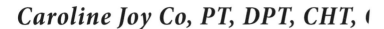
Caroline Joy Co, PT, DPT, CHT,

Myofascial Trigger Point Release of the

Upper Extremity

A Review of Current Research

Myofascial Trigger Point Release of the Upper Extremity

ISBN: 1451598343
EAN-13: 9781451598346
Printed in the United States of America

Disclaimer:
This book is intended for informational and educational purposes only. It is not meant to provide any medical advice. Many of the product names referred to herein are trademarks or registered trademarks of their respective owners. Care has been taken to confirm the accuracy of the information presented and to describe generally accepted practices. However, the authors, editors, and publisher are not responsible for errors or omissions or for any consequences from application of the information in this book and make no warranty, expressed or implied, with respect to the currency, completeness, or accuracy of the contents of the publication. Application of this information in a particular situation remains the professional responsibility of the practitioner.

Rehabsurge, Inc.'s mission is to support healthcare and education professionals to continue their educational and professional development. Rehabsurge is committed to identifying, promoting, and implementing innovative continuing education activities that can increase and impart professional knowledge and skills through books, audiobooks, or digital e-books based on sound scientific and clinically derived research. The first Rehabsurge continuing education book was published in July 2009.

As a sponsor of Continuing Education (CE) seminars and workshops, we enable professionals to enhance their skills, pursue professional interests, and redefine their specialties within their respective disciplines while earning CEUs, CE credits, or Contact Hours. Offerings include CE books, audiobooks, and digital e-books, all of which are focused on the latest treatment and assessment approaches and include discussions of alternative and state-of-the art therapies.
Rehabsurge exists to provide the latest treatment and assessment approaches to the practicing clinician. The basic proposition of our business is simple, solid, and timeless. When we bring the latest knowledge and skill to our clients, we successfully nurture and protect our brand. That is the key to fulfilling our ultimate obligation to provide consistently attractive books, audiobooks, and digital e-books.

For permissions and additional information contact us:
Rehabsurge, Inc.
PO Box 287 Baldwin, NY 11510.
Phone: +1 (516) 515-1267
Email: ceu@rehabsurge.com

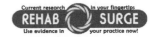

DISABILITY POLICY:

Rehabsurge seeks to ensure that all students have access to its activities. To that end, it is committed to providing support services and assistance for equal access for learners with disabilities. Rehabsurge has a firm commitment to meeting the guidelines of the Americans with Disabilities Act and Section 504 of the Rehabilitation Act of 1973. Rehabsurge will provide support services and assistance for students with disabilities, including reasonable accommodations, modifications, and appropriate services to all learners with documented disabilities.

About the Author

Caroline Joy Co, PT, DPT, CHT, CSFA, is a licensed physical therapist and certified hand therapist whose clinical experience includes acute, subacute, home health, and outpatient settings. Her background includes Community-Based Therapy that is designed to help people with disabilities access therapy in their communities. She is the President and CEO of PTSponsor.com, an online resource for U.S. hospitals and clinics that seek to sponsor and hire foreign-trained rehabilitation therapists. She specializes in hand therapy through an integrated approach that includes education, counsel, and exercise. She is also certified in functional assessment for work hardening and work conditioning.

Co is also the President of Rehabsurge, a continuing education company and a contracting agency. Her past affiliations include Long Beach Medical Center, Horizon Health and Subacute Center, and Grandell Therapy and Nursing Center.

Co was a professional speaker for Summit Professional Education, Cross Country Education and Dogwood Institute. She received her transitional doctorate from A.T. Still University and her BS in Physical Therapy from University of the Philippines College of Allied Medical Professions. She is licensed in California, Nevada, and New York.

Full Disclosure

To comply with professional boards/associations standards, all planners, speakers, and reviewers involved in the development of continuing education content are required to disclose their relevant financial relationships. An individual has a relevant financial relationship if he or she has a financial relationship in any amount occurring in the last 12 months, with any commercial interest whose products or services are discussed in their presentation content over which the individual has control. Relevant financial relationships must be disclosed to the audience.

As part of its accreditation with boards/associations, Rehabsurge, Inc. is required to "resolve" any reported conflicts of interest prior to the educational activity. The presentation will be scientifically balanced and free of commercial bias or influence.

To comply with professional boards/associations standards:

I declare that neither I nor my family has any financial relationship in any amount occurring in the last 12 months, with a commercial interest whose products or services are discussed in my presentation. Additionally all planners involved do not have any financial relationship.

Caroline Joy Co, PT, DPT, CHT, CSFA

Course Description

This course will teach myofascial trigger point release concepts. By utilizing the trigger point techniques, patients make rapid improvement in their status. Outcomes have reflected reduced therapy sessions with permanent improvement as well as the patient's ability to self-manage their condition with the home exercise programs. Methods for locating and deactivating trigger points using a variety of techniques and modalities will be explored. After reading the book, you will be able to use these techniques immediately upon return to your practice.

Myofascial release involves sustained pressure and graded stretch applied to the soft tissue, which is guided entirely by the feedback obtained from the patient's body. The feedback felt by the therapist while applying the stretch determines the direction of the stretch, its duration, and the amount of force applied. From shoulder disorders to elbow injuries to debilitating hand and wrist problems, quicker improvement and more favorable outcomes are unquestionably dependent on proper rehabilitation technique and individualized, forward thinking concepts, and application. What were previously considered complementary therapeutic methods are now proven, evidence-based techniques and modalities that care for the total patient and are imperative for today's therapist.

Myofascial release can benefit individuals of almost all age groups; the release of the muscle tightness (as a result of fascial involvement) facilitates the maximal elongation of the muscles, leading to a decrease in the constant pull being experienced by the tendons and other associated structures.

Course Objectives

1. Demonstrate how to identify and correct for the most common factors that precipitate and perpetuate myofascial trigger points.

2. Identify techniques for deactivating trigger points including trigger point pressure release and myofascial release.

3. Interpret client history and assessment findings to ascertain irritability.

4. Utilize self-care techniques for deactivating trigger points.

5. Demonstrate trigger point palpation using STAR palpation.

6. Apply strain-counterstrain techniques and integrated neuromuscular inhibition techniques to deactivate trigger points.

Table of contents/Course Outline

Introduction

Fascia refers to an embryonic tissue component of the connective tissue system that covers the human body. Fascia is noted to interpenetrate between various tissues and other structures and is generally present around the muscles, bones, organs, nerves, blood vessels, and other structures. Fascia can be also referred to as an uninterrupted, three-dimensional web of tissue that extends in, on, and around almost all structures in the human body. Some of the important functions served by the fascia include maintaining structural integrity, providing support and protection, and acting as a shock absorber (Simons et al, 1999).

Any kind of trauma, micro or macro, chronic or acute, can cause mal-alignment and contraction of the fascia along with the associated muscles as protective reaction to the trauma. However, such mal-alignment can result in a significant amount of strain, leading to a number of cascading events such as loss of adaptive capacity of the muscles, loss of flexibility in the muscles, lack of muscle spontaneity, pain, and limitation of movement (Travell & Simons, 1983).

The fascia covers the muscles at different levels including at the fibril and microfibril levels. Therefore, the fascia has a vital role in deciding the length and function of the muscles, and any factors affecting the myofascial tissues will inadvertently have an effect on muscle function (Schleip et al, 2005).

Myofascial trigger point therapy plays an important role in the diagnosis and treatment of the conditions affecting the myofascial tissues. Inappropriate fascial strains can result from a wide variety of conditions including physical trauma, inflammatory processes, or structural imbalances. Myofascial release can be employed to loosen or release the tightness in connective tissues (or the fascia). Myofascial release involves sustained pressure and graded stretch applied to the soft tissue, which is guided entirely by the feedback obtained from the patient's body. The feedback felt by the therapist while applying the stretch determines the direction of the stretch, its duration, and the amount of force applied (Hans & Harrison, 1997).

Myofascial release can benefit individuals of almost all age groups; the release of the muscle tightness (as a result of fascial involvement) facilitates the maximal elongation of the muscles, leading to a decrease in the constant pull being experienced by the tendons and other associated structures (Jacobs & Walls, 1997).

Brief history and some definitions

The oldest known documents that discuss sensitive areas on the skin and the tender points on the human body belongs to the Chinese and the Japanese books of ancient medicine . These discussed the concepts of energy meridians and acupuncture, some of which even date back to the time of Hippocrates (400 BC). Sources say that during the 19th century, Froriep identified that certain tender, tight cords or bands within a muscle were responsible for production of pain in the muscles. Although there were many other researchers who discussed similar concepts, it was not until late 1940s that the term "myofascial" begin to appear in medical literature through the works of Travell, Gorell, and many others. The first complete publication that talked about the concept of specific trigger points, referred pain, and a thorough review of the other published literature was brought out by Travell and Simons in 1983. Travell and Simons are therefore considered the pioneers

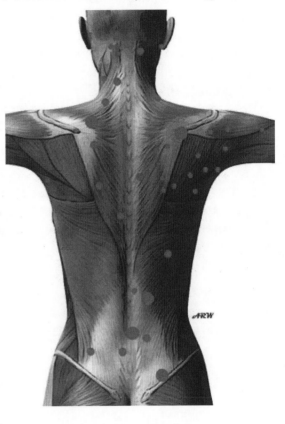

in the area of myofascial trigger point syndrome. Since then, many others have published several studies and books regarding the concept of myofascial trigger point syndrome and other related concepts (Lavell et al, 2007).

Some common definitions:

Analgesia: the absence of pain in response to a stimulation that would normally be painful (Cyriax, 1984)

Allodynia: condition where pain is caused by a stimulus that does not normally provoke pain (Cyriax, 1984)

Causalgia: a syndrome of sustained burning pain, allodynia, and hyperpathia after a traumatic nerve lesion; now classified as complex regional pain syndrome II (Cyriax, 1984)

Dysthesia: unpleasant abnormal sensation (Cyriax, 1984)

Hyperesthesia: increased sensitivity to stimulation, excluding the special senses (Cyriax, 1984)

Hyperpathia: an abnormally painful reaction to a stimulus usually caused by a repetitive stimulus (Cyriax, 1984)

Hyperalgesia: an increased pain response to a stimulus that is normally painful (Cyriax, 1984)

Hypoalgesia: diminished pain in response to a normally painful stimulus (Cyriax, 1984)

Pain: an unpleasant sensory and emotional experience associated with actual or potential tissue damage (Cyriax, 1984)

Anatomy of a skeletal muscle

A muscle is a collection of muscle cells or fibers. The muscles are covered by and protected by a layer of connective fascia tissue often referred to as epimysium. This tissue is continuous with the connective tissue that surrounds each muscle fiber, tendon, bone, and nerve vessel. The muscles are further subdivided into fascicles, which is a bundle of muscle fibers called myofibers or myocytes. Myofibers or myocytes can be further subdivided into myofibril or fibrils. The myofibrils are mainly composed of certain individual proteins known as thin and thick myofilaments (Grieve, 1986).

Within the muscle are the sarcomeres and sarcoplasmic retinaculum, which encircle the myofibrils. Sarcomere is the contractile or functional unit of muscle, while sarcoplasmic retinaculum refers to the part of a muscle cell that produces energy. The sarcomere is the smallest unit of a muscle or a cell and is the functional unit of length in a muscle. The sarcomere contains proteins known as myosin and actin. They account for the bands present in the sarcomere. The orderly overlapping of these two proteins actin and myosin cause the striated appearance of light and dark bands found on cardiac and skeletal muscles (Janda, 1993).

The A band is the dark band and corresponds to the length of a bundle of myosin filaments. The A bands are then dissected into a somewhat lighter area known as the H zone. During muscle contraction, actin slides over the myosin and encroaches into the H zone so that the H zone shortens to a certain extent. In the middle of the H zone, a dark band known as the M line—comprised of certain protein fibers that help in anchoring the myosin filaments—may also be noted (Melzack & Wall, 1988).

The light bands are known as I bands, which are bisected by a protein disc known as Z lines. The I bands, A bands, and Z lines overlap each other during muscle contractions. The A band for the most part does not move. This is an important finding. Because the A band generally corresponds to the length of the myosin filaments, and these filaments do not shorten, the width of the A band also does not shorten (Melzack & Wall, 1988).

Three main events occur when a muscle contracts. These include: electrical excitation of a muscle fiber, excitation-contraction coupling, and muscle fiber contraction.

Electrical excitation

The muscle fibers (or cells) are generally stimulated by a nerve cell (motor neuron), which results in depolarization (change in the polarity) of the sarcolemma. When this process reaches a certain limit—commonly referred to as the threshold level—an electrical signal known as action potential is generated (DiGiovanna, 2005).

Excitation-contraction coupling

The transmission of action potential causes calcium ions to be released from the sarcoplasmic retinaculum. The calcium ions released couple electrical excitation to muscle fiber contraction by binding to a regulatory protein called troponin, which is attached to the actin filament and another regulatory protein called tropomyosin. The binding of calcium to troponin results in a change in its shape, which pulls tropomyosin away from the myosin-binding sites on the actin filament.

Muscle fiber contraction

The pulling away from the myosin-binding site leads to the exposure of the actin filament, which leads to muscle contraction. A muscle fiber contracts due to actin filaments sliding past the myosin filaments. Each muscle fiber is shortened by about 1% of its resting length during each contraction cycle. The muscle fiber returns to its resting length when the contraction cycle is completed.

Some of the important steps in the contraction cycle include:

1. ATP hydrolysis

2. Attachment of myosin to actin to form cross-bridges

3. Power stroke

4. Detachment of myosin from actin

The contraction cycle continues until the calcium levels within the muscle cells remain high. As the intracellular calcium levels drop, the process is reversed and the muscle fiber relaxes (East Tennessee State University, 2001).

Types of muscle contraction

Three types of muscle contraction have been described in a clinical setting.

Isometric contraction:

The muscle contracts or moves in a specified direction which is matched by the practitioner's effort in the opposite direction so that no movement is allowed to take place (East Tennessee State University, 2001).

Concentric isotonic contraction:

The muscle contracts or moves in a specified direction. The practitioner's counterforce is less than that of the patient so that movement is allowed to take place in the patient's intended direction (East Tennessee State University, 2001).

Eccentric isotonic contraction:

The muscle contracts or moves in a specified direction. The practitioner's counterforce is greater than that of the patient so that movement is allowed to take place in the patient's opposite direction. The muscle lengthens when the patient is trying to shorten the muscle (East Tennessee State University, 2001).

Concentric contraction

Concentric contractions occur against resistance. It allows toning and strengthening of the weakened musculature involved in contraction. The affected muscle is allowed to contract, with some resistance from the practitioner. The patient's force is greater than the practitioner's resistance. The patient builds his force slowly, not with sudden maximal effort. The practitioner maintains a constant degree of resistance. The use of weights during exercise is an example of concentric contraction (East Tennessee State University, 2001).

Eccentric contraction

The muscle to be stretched is contracted by the patient and is prevented from doing so by the practitioner, by means of superior therapist effort, so that the contraction is rapidly overcome and reversed, introducing stretch into the contracting muscle. The process should take no more than four seconds. Origin and insertion do not approximate. The muscle should be stretched to full physiological resting length. The therapist's force is greater than that of the patient. Less than maximal patient force should be employed at first. Subsequent contractions build towards this if discomfort is not excessive. Avoid using eccentric contractions on head and neck muscles if the patient is frail, very pain-sensitive, or osteoporotic. The patient should anticipate soreness for several days in the affected muscles. Most closed chain exercises use eccentric contraction (East Tennessee State University, 2001).

Laws affecting muscle tissues

There are several laws that can explain the effect of different factors on the muscle tissues. These can give an insight of the cause, mechanism of action, and the ways to treat problems affecting the muscles.

Wolff's law: biological systems deform in relation to the lines of force impressed on them. A good example for Wolff's law would be astronauts in space. Because their bones are not subjected to the lines of gravity, they lose bone density (O'Sullivan & Siegelman, 2010).

Hooke's law: deformation imposed on the elastic body is proportional to the stress placed on it

Newton's third law: For every action, there is an equal and opposite reaction. When a patient falls, the injured tissues will shorten and the opposing structures will lengthen. Any attempt to stretch the area will be resisted (O'Sullivan & Siegelman, 2010).

A myofascial trigger point is a hyperirritable spot, present usually within a taut band of skeletal muscle, which is painful on compression and can give rise to a characteristic referred pain, motor dysfunction, and autonomic phenomena. These trigger points can be found in the muscle that originates in the vicinity of dysfunctional endplates (nerve junctions or muscle to nerve connection points). These are palpable as taut bands and are associated with other features such as nodularity and limited range of motion (Fleckenstein, 2009).

Trigger points associated with myofascial and visceral pain often lies within the areas of referred pain, but many are located at a distance from them. Brief, intense stimulation of trigger points frequently produces prolonged relief of pain (Fleckenstein, 2009).

Mechanism of injury

These trigger points are commonly formed following repetitive movement, high velocity movements, or holding the muscles in stressful positions for prolonged periods of time. Several other types of trigger points include cutaneous, fascial, ligamentous, and periosteal (Gerwin, 2005).

Myofascial trigger point regions were demonstrated to have strong (93.3%) anatomic correspondences with classical acupuncture points. They also had 97% correlation for treating pain conditions and over 93% correlation in treating somatovisceral conditions (Gerwin, 2005).

Myofascial Trigger points

The incidence of myofascial pain syndrome with associated trigger points appears to vary between 30 and 85% of people presenting to pain clinics, and the condition is more prevalent in women than in men. Patients often complain of persistent pain in certain specific regions. The pain can vary in intensity. It is most frequently found in regions such as the head, neck, shoulders, extremities, and lower back. Pain may be localized to certain specific regions that are painful when pressed. In some instances, the trigger points can transmit or activate pain sensations some distance away from themselves in target tissues. When not actively referring or radiating, they are noted to remain latent (Lundon, 2003).

Clinical Symptoms

A trigger point is a localized tender hardening in a skeletal muscle. This is a region of hyper-irritability in a muscle or is a localized spot of tenderness. Microtrauma (overload) or macrotrauma (sudden high velocity movement) can give rise to the formation of trigger points. The affected individuals often complain of referred pain along with occasional experiences of burning sensation in the affected regions or trigger points. Some of the substances that are found in high concentration in these are include bradykinin, prostaglandin, and hydrogen ions (Gross, 1992).

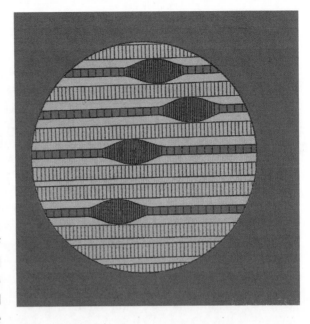

Referred pain pattern is often misleading and may lead to false treatment in many instances. The activation of trigger points can lead to the projection of pain at a region far away from the trigger point. It becomes critical to identify the right trigger point, and pathways of pain distribution to clearly identify the affected regions while ruling out the possibility of injuries in the regions where pain is elicited or referred (Gross, 1992).

Patients suffering from myofascial pain syndromes often have certain autonomic and proprioceptive disturbances, such as increased sweating and salivation or a positive pilomotor reflex (occurrence of goose bumps). Other symptoms associated with trigger points include edema and cellulite formation, dermatomal hair loss, and sleep disturbances (Gross, 1992).

When a contraction requires 70% of available strength of the affected muscle, blood flow is reduced and oxygen availability diminishes in the muscle housing the trigger point. Our bodies compensate until the adaptive tissues are exhausted. Decompensation begins, and symptoms such as pain, restriction, and limited ROM become apparent (Gross, 1992).

Physical Findings

There are several physical findings that can be elicited in patients with trigger points. Muscle fibers that house a trigger point are taut, giving a rope-like sensation when palpated. They have overshortened sarcomeres along with overstretched areas. They may also have tender and painful nodules. Increased pressure on the nodules of the affected muscles will elicit referred pain patterns. Patient pain recognition is considered as an essential criterion for the identification or confirmation of a trigger point. The patient can experience pain when the said trigger point is compressed or on needle insertion. Other physical findings associated with myofascial trigger points include local twitch response, limited range of motion (ROM), muscle weakness, and a positive stretch sign (pain develops in the joint during myofascial stretching) (Eastwood et al, 1998).

Classification of Myofascial Trigger Points

The myofascial trigger points have been classified in several ways. Below is one of the frequently used in the majority published literatures and in clinical practice.

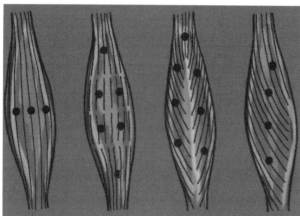

Myofascial trigger points can be classified as:

Active—tender and produce spontaneous pain without digital compression (Shah et al, 2003)

Latent—silent, does not cause spontaneous pain, but is tender upon palpation (Shah et al, 2003)

Satellite—develops near the primary point; resolves once the main trigger point is resolved (Shah et al, 2003)

Central—present near the center of the muscle fibers and is closely associated with dysfunctional endplates (Shah et al, 2003)

Attachment—located at the osseous attachment of the muscle (Shah et al, 2003)

CHAPTER 3 DIAGNOSIS OF MYOFASCIAL TRIGGER POINT SYNDROME

The diagnosis of myofascial trigger points can be quite challenging. A proper knowledge of the muscle anatomy and physiology becomes quite essential while evaluating a patient for myofascial trigger point syndrome. Below is a step by step approach to arrive at the diagnosis.

History

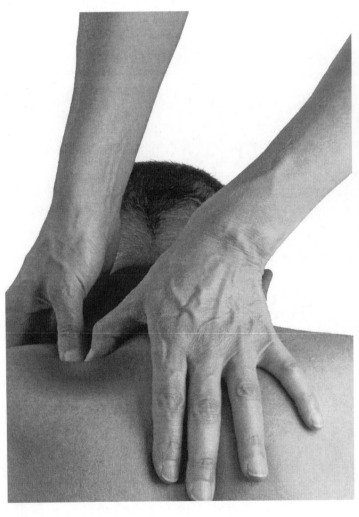

There is often a history of trauma or overload associated with the trigger points. Major injuries or sudden high velocity movement are often remembered. Microtrauma results from constant overloading of the muscles is often ignored by the patient. Thereby, it becomes important for you to inquire about the profession, and the associated factors such as repeated muscle movements, improper posture or stressful jobs. Additionally, quality of life also needs to be assessed.

Diagnostic Criteria for myofascial trigger points

1. Look for tenderness in a palpable taut band or nodule.

• The patient will recognize the pain evoked by pressure on the tender spot. This primary criterion is called "Spot tenderness of the nodule in a palpable tight band".

2. Palpate taut bands and identify nodules. An acronym is used to denote the steps for early diagnosis of trigger points.

STAR palpation
Sensitivity (or 'Tenderness')
Tissue texture change
Asymmetry – There will be a muscle imbalance causing asymmetry.
Range of motion reduced – The muscles will not be able to reach their normal resting length, or joints may have a restricted range·

3. Establish referred pain pattern.

During the physical examination, the referred pain pattern for the involved trigger point must be established with digital compression of the active trigger point. The region or the pattern of referred pain may vary in each patient and also based on the severity of the condition.

4. Establish diagnosis

Palpation is critical in the identification of the trigger point. Three methods have been described for trigger point palpation-- flat palpation, pincer palpation, and deep palpation.

The **flat palpation** is when you palpate a trigger point using the thumb or fingers that are held flat. The skin is pushed to one side, and the finger is drawn across the muscle fibers. You should follow the involved fiber in a distal direction and

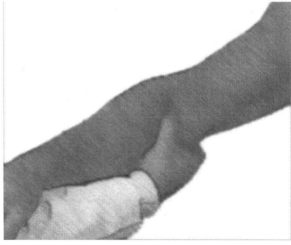

in a proximal direction. Then, apply
the pressure. A taut band may be felt
passing under your finger. Snapping
palpation, like plucking of a violin, is
used to identify the specific trigger
point.

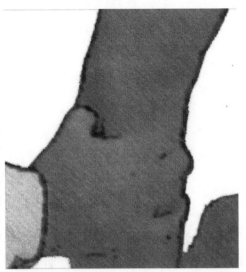

The **pincer palpation**
technique is when you would grab the
affected area with the trigger point in
it and hold it. The pinching action is
used to apply the pressure. The fibers
are pressed between the fingers in a
rolling manner while attempting to
locate a taut band.

Deep palpation may be used to find a trigger point that is obscured
by superficial tissue over the involved region. The fingertip is placed over
the muscle attachment of the area suspected of housing the trigger point.
When the patient's symptoms are reproduced by pressing onto the area, a
trigger point may be presumed to be located.

Pointers
- Muscles which contain trigger points will often hurt when contracted.
- Myofascial Trigger Points are areas of increased energy consumption
and lowered oxygen supply.
- They cannot reach their normal resting length.
- Referred pain is caused by the brain mislocating the messages.
- Self perpetuating, will never go away unless adequately treated.

Differential Diagnosis

It is important to understand the cause of the patient's problems. O'Sullivan
et al (2010), have compiled a list of special tests and clinical presentations.
These conditions can also produce myofascial trigger points. However,
differential diagnosis is important to know the cause of the problem and
provide the most appropriate care.

Acromioclavicular Joint (sprain, subluxation or dislocation)

Patient will complain of : Pain and instability noted with abduction

The onset of the injury is : Due to overhead activity; trauma; fall on tip of shoulder or outstretched arm

Physical Exam : Local pain experienced last 30° > 90° or with horizontal adduction; Local swelling; step-off appearance with dependent arm holding weight; Painful arc in abduction, increase in joint play

Special Tests: Horizontal adduction humerus

Biceps Tendonitis

Patient will complain of : Local snapping sensation over bicipital groove, pain

The onset of the injury is : After activity or repetitive training, ages 45 – 65, more common in females

Physical Exam : Local anterior tenderness, chronic pain at proximal arm, symptoms worse with abduction and external rotation; arm held close to side of body; Resisted elbow flexion and supination increases pain

Special Tests: Yergason's test

Calcific Supraspinatus Tendonitis

Patient will complain of : Severe, disabling pain

The onset of the injury is : Acute, fulminating attack

Physical Exam : Intense pain in deltoid region, rapid increase in severity, no relief with rest; Swelling, arm held in protective adduction; Painful arc from 60°- 120°

Special Tests: Impingement tests; Calcium deposits seen on x-ray, sclerosis, cystic changes

Degenerative Supraspinatus Tendonitis

Patient will complain of : Low-grade ache

Physical Exam : Local, lateral pain and tenderness that increase with abduction; worse at night; Crepitus over supraspinatus tendon; Decrease ROM

Special Tests: Impingement tests

Frozen Shoulder

Patient will complain of : Painfully restricted shoulder motion

The onset of the injury is : Insidious or due to precipitating factors

Physical Exam: Initial pain during activity and rest in deltoid with progression to stiffness; Patient protective of arm, motion is guarded;   Movement

limited in capsular pattern decrease in joint play, girdle hunching
Special Tests: Arthrography reveals reduced joint volume

GH Dislocation Subluxation

Patient will complain of : Sensation of catching or lose control with subluxation, complete loss of functions with dislocation
The onset of the injury is : Forced abduction and ER, fall on extended arm
Physical Exam : Severe pain and disability with acute dislocation; Square appearance; reduced and increased anterior glide in chronic cases
Special Tests: Apprehension test, Hill-Sachs lesion noted on x-ray if recurrent

Rotator Cuff Lesions

Patient will complain of : Catching sensation at 90°
The onset of the injury is : Traumatic rupture; mild trauma if tendon degenerated
Physical Exam : Pain with rotation or abduction, can't sleep on involved side; Atrophy; palpable cleft with rupture; Unable to resist abduction
Special Tests: Drop arm test; with arthrography will see leakage of dye into bursa

Normal

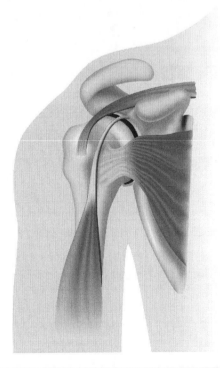

Rotator cuff problems

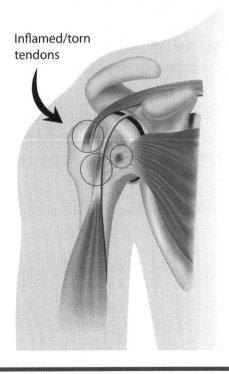

Inflamed/torn tendons

Subacromial Bursitis

Patient will complain of : Painful to abduction

The onset of the injury is : Acute, within 2-3 days of strenuous activity or immobilization

Physical Exam : Severe, local tenderness, hard to distinguish from supraspinatus tendonitis; Lateral swelling; Painful arc from 60°- 120°

Special Tests: Impingement tests

Thoracic Outlet Syndrome

Patient will complain of : Paresthesias and hyperesthesias in medial arm, pain, swelling, cyanosis, cold limb

The onset of the injury is: scalene spasm, or hypertrophy, clavicular drooping; congenital anomalies

Physical Exam : Pain and sensory changes related to position or activity; Rounded, sagging shoulder posture; Weakness in C8, T1 muscles

Special Tests: Adson, costoclavicular, hyperabduction, elevated arm stress test, decreased sensation in C8, T1 distribution

The Brachial Plexus

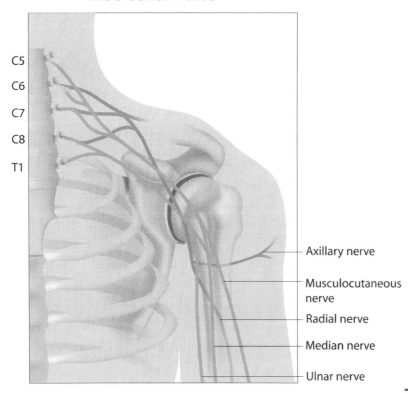

C5
C6
C7
C8
T1

Axillary nerve

Musculocutaneous nerve

Radial nerve

Median nerve

Ulnar nerve

Bursitis Non-inflammatory (Olecranon)

Patient will complain of : Lump
The onset of the injury is : Direct trauma or repetitive stress
Physical Exam : Painless; Cystic swelling; Dislocation (Posterior)

Dislocation

Patient will complain of : Incapacitating pain and deformity
The onset of the injury is : Fall on outstretched hand or severe hyperextension
Physical Exam : Pain, loss of function; associated soft tissue injury; Deformity or swelling; Loss of motion is a late complication
Special Tests: Olecranon palpated posteriorly

Intraarticular Fracture

Patient will complain of : Pain, swelling, deformity
The onset of the injury is : Blow to flexed elbow or longitudinal loading to extended elbow
Physical Exam : Pain and dysfunction; Disruption of isosceles triangle; Loss of motion is a late complication
Special Tests: Radiography

Olecranon Fracture

Patient will complain of : Pain, swelling, deformity
The onset of the injury is : Direct trauma or triceps avulsion
Physical Exam : Pain and dysfunction; Disruption of isosceles triangle; Loss of motion is a late complication
Special Tests: Radiography

Radial Head Fracture

Patient will complain of : Pain, swelling, deformity
The onset of the injury is : Axial load on pronated forearm or valgus compression
Physical Exam : Pain and dysfunction; Lateral swelling from hemarthrosis and disruption of lateral triangle; Loss of motion is a late complication
Special Tests: Radiography

Supracondylar Fracture

Patient will complain of : Pain, swelling, deformity
The onset of the injury is : Fall on outstretched hand
Physical Exam : Neurovascular compromise; Posterior displacement of

distal fragment; Loss of motion is a late complication
Special Tests: Radiography; fat pad sign

Lateral Epicondylitis
Patient will complain of : Dull or sharp lateral pain
The onset of the injury is : Insidious, overuse
Physical Exam : Swelling, pain weakness of wrist extension and grip; Lateral swelling
Special Tests: Decreased wrist extensor and grip strength

Myositis Ossificans
Patient will complain of : Painful swelling of brachialis muscle
The onset of the injury is : Direct muscle trauma or secondary to fracture or dislocation
Physical Exam : Rapidly enlarging painful mass; Mass in muscle or soft tissue; Limited motion
Special Tests: Well-circumscribed osseous mass

Nurse-maids' (Pulled) Elbow
Patient will complain of : Pain localized to superior radioulnar joint
The onset of the injury is : Longitudinal full on forearm
Physical Exam : Avoids use of arm; Arm held in pronation; Inability to supinate without pain
Special Tests: Palpate sulcus proximal to radial head

Volkmann's Contracture
Patient will complain of : Severe pain in forearm; sensation of pressure if compartment syndrome
The onset of the injury is : Nerve and muscle ischemia, secondary to arterial compromise
Physical Exam : Pain within 2 hours increased by passive finger extension; pallor; paresis; pulselessness; Wrist extension and finger flexion contractures; Paralysis and contractures are late complications

Bacterial Arthritis
Patient will complain of : Pain at rest, exacerbated by movement
The onset of the injury is : May occur after bites, wounds, or septicemia
Physical Exam : Local pain, swelling and redness; tender to palpation; Swelling of involved joints; Movement restricted by pain and swelling
Special Tests: Joint aspiration

Osteoarthritis

Patient will complain of : Painful, nodular swelling of DIPs

The onset of the injury is : Insidious in the elderly

Physical Exam : Local pain and tenderness; Deforming bony protuberances on dorsum of DIPs (Heberden's nodes) rarely on PIPs; Instability of involved joints

Special Tests: Radiography

Rheumatoid Arthritis

Patient will complain of : Painful swelling in wrist, MP, and PIP joints

The onset of the injury is : Insidious, common in women aged 20-40

Physical Exam : Pain, swelling and redness in joints tendon sheath inflammation; morning stiffness exacerbations and remissions; Deformities (e.g. swan neck, ulnar drift, MPs, boutonniere); Instability and muscle imbalance

Special Tests: RA factor, ESR, radiography, Bunnell-Littler and functional tests

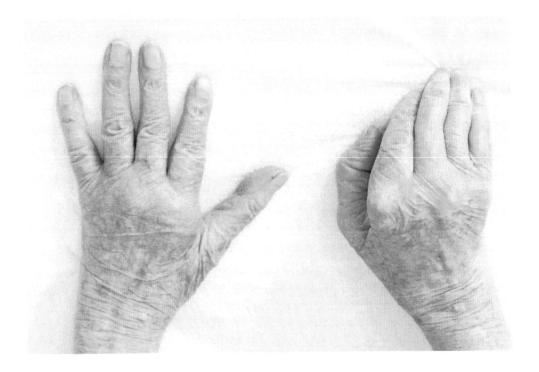

Carpal Tunnel Syndrome

Patient will complain of : Numbness, pain or paresthesia on radial side palm
The onset of the injury is : Insidious, ages 40-60
Physical Exam : Sensory changes aggravated by prolonged use of hand, is worse at night; Thenar atrophy; Weakness in pinch
Special Tests: Phalen's test, Tinel's sign, Nerve Conduction Velocity test

DeQuervain's Disease

Patient will complain of : Tenderness over radial styloid
The onset of the injury is : Direct trauma or repetitive minor irritation
Physical Exam : Pain produced by active thumb abduction or passive stretch of extensor pollicis brevis and abductor pollicus longus; Tendon sheath swelling; Weakness of thumb abduction
Special Tests: Finkelstein's test

Dupuytren's Contracture

Patient will complain of : Palmar nodule or contracture
The onset of the injury is : Insidious, most common in men aged 40 -60
Physical Exam : Painless fibrosis of palmar aponeurosis; Flexion contractures in digits 4 & 5 secondary to palmar contracture; Inability to extend digits
Special Tests: Contracture initially demonstrated by constant length principle

Kienbock's Disease

Patient will complain of : Wrist pain
The onset of the injury is : Trauma-related in adults
Physical Exam : Pain increased by wrist flexion and extension, lunate tender to palpation, Progressive limitation of wrist motion
Special Tests: Radiography

Peripheral Nerve Compression

Patient will complain of : Weakness and sensory changes
The onset of the injury is : Trauma or insidious
Physical Exam : Sensory or motor loss; varies depending on severity of nerve damage; Deformities (e.g. ape hand, wrist drop); Weakness in muscles involved
Special Tests: Nerve conduction velocity test, manual muscle test

Myofascial release refers to the use of sustained pressure to loosen or release tightness in connective tissues (fascia). The use of pressure has many advantages such as relaxing the contracted muscles, increasing blood circulation and venous, and lymphatic drainage in the affected regions (Imamura, 1997).

The myofascial release techniques are directed towards the non-dynamic connective tissue component of soft tissues. Such tissue is slow to shorten; it requires a lengthy period of applied load (Imamura, 1997).

Trigger Point Acupuncture or Dry Needling

Dry needling is the use of a solid needle for deactivation and desensitization of a myofascial trigger point, which should stimulate a healing response in that

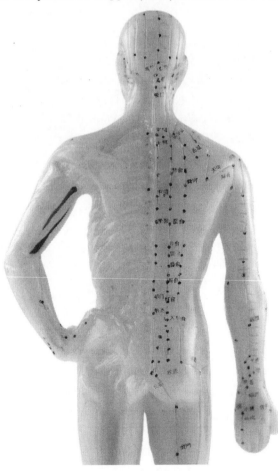

tissue and reduce the biomechanical stress of the muscle treated. Also known as intramuscular stimulation, dry needling is a physical intervention that uses dry needles to stimulate trigger points, diagnose, and treat neuromuscular pain and functional movement deficits (Fleckenstein, 2009).

There is substantial peer-reviewed medical literature on intramuscular stimulation. Dry needling is within the scope of practice of physical therapists in Colorado, South Carolina, Georgia, Maryland, New Hampshire, Virginia, Texas, Nevada, and New Mexico. Professor Melzack states the nearly 80% of trigger points are in exactly the same positions known as acupuncture points (Fleckenstein, 2009).

Acupuncture originates in Europe and Asia and has been practiced for centuries. There are a few differences between acupuncture and myofascial trigger points. One of them is stretching, because acupuncture does not follow up with stretching while for myofascial trigger point, stretching is extremely important (Fleckenstein, 2009).

Some of the differences between trigger point dry needling and acupuncture are:

Clinical Application:

Dry needling assesses and treats myofascial pain due to myofascial trigger points.

Acupuncture diagnoses and treats several pathological conditions including visceral and systemic dysfunction.

Follow up treatment:

Dry needling follows with myofascial stretching exercises.

Acupuncture has no stretching or anything similar.

Needling Technique:

Dry needling use one needle inserted in the myofascial trigger points.

Acupuncture uses multiple needles.

Vapocoolant Spray

Travell and Simons (1983) considered the use of passive stretching of the affected muscle after application of sprayed vapocoolant as the "single most effective treatment" for trigger point pain. The application of a vapocoolant spray requires three sweeps 8–12 inches on the skin above the trigger point to referred pain pattern, then below the trigger point to referred pain pattern. This is followed by a gentle stretch. This procedure is normally repeated until full range of motion of the muscle group is achieved. A maximum of three repetitions can be done before rewarming the area with moist heat. Prolonged exposure to the vapocoolant spray must be avoided by ensuring that each spray pass lasts less than six seconds. Patients must also be instructed not to overstretch muscles after a spray and stretch therapy session.

Modalities for Trigger Point Release

There are several modalities that can be utilized as pre-treatment techniques to the affected muscle.

1. Hot packs

Heat can help elongate and improve the extensibility of the structures housing the trigger point. Moist heat when applied for 15 to 20 minutes aids in muscle relaxation (Prentice, 1994).

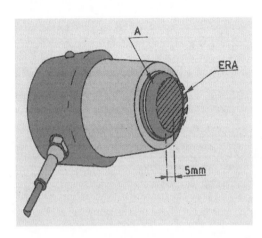

2. Ultrasound

Pulsed or continuous ultrasound are both effective in reducing myofascial pain (Prentice, 1994).

3. Myofascial Stretching

Myofascial stretching refers to passive stretch for more than 30 seconds. This is performed at a slow rate. Place the muscle in stretched position where tensions are sensed, and then allow the muscle to relax. Slow delayed persistent change in the muscle occurs in response to continuously applied load. Stretching should be gentle in order to lengthen overshortened sarcomeres. We must stretch the muscle to bring the muscle to an ergonomically correct state (Beaulieu, 1981).

4. Progressive Pressure or Ischemic Compression

The clinician helps the muscle relax by deactivating the trigger point via progressive pressure. Trigger Point Pressure Release is the repeated applications of moderate pressure (5 seconds each application). It is applied slowly. The clinician should pause at least 2–3 seconds before applying pressure again. Ischemic compression is the application of sustained pressure for at least 30 seconds to 2 minutes.

Myofascial Stretching

There are different variations noted in the standard stretching techniques.

- Contract relax Antagonist contract: Strong isometric contractions of the antagonist muscle is followed by active stretching by the patient (Voss et al, 1985).

- Proprioceptive Neuromuscular Facilitation (PNF) variations including hold-relax and contract relax (Voss et al, 1985).

- Active isolated stretching: uses active stretching by the patient and reciprocal inhibition mechanisms. Precise localization of the muscle that needs to be stretched is identified. Repetitive fairly short duration, isotonic muscle contractions are performed to produce relaxation. Then, the muscle is stretched just beyond the point of light irritation. Repetitions continue until adequate gain in the muscle length is achieved (Mattes, 1995).

- Yoga stretching (and static stretching): Adopting specific postures based on traditional yoga and maintaining these for some time with deep relaxation breathing. It is a form of self-induced viscoelastic myofascial release (Galantino et al, 2004).

- Ballistic stretching: stretching by using rapid and bouncing movements. There is a risk of irritation or injury.

- Muscle energy technique: utilizes the assumed effect of reduced tone experienced by the muscle after brief periods of isometric contraction.

Precautions and Contraindications

Deep myofascial therapy, massage, stretching, and releases are uncomfortable. Myofascial trigger points release can be exquisitely painful. Scar releases have been described as having surgery without anesthesia. However, the treatment administered may hurt but "feels good" at the same time. Beneficial hurt should not exceed the patient's physical and/or emotional pain limit (McAtee & Charland, 1999).

Trigger point release therapy is not advised or should be practiced with caution in consultation with the patient's physician under following circumstances:
- Malignancy
- Open wounds
- Severe arteriosclerosis
- Aneurysm
- Subdural hematoma
- Advanced Osteoporosis (bone loses density)
- Anticoagulant therapy (bruises easily)

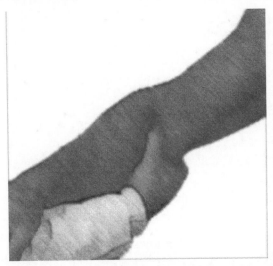

If your patient is on glucose-lowering mediation, you should test the blood glucose level prior to treatment and immediately following treatment to prevent dangerous hypoglycemia. Also, deep pressure therapy can lower blood pressure. Keep your patient lying down (horizontal) for 20 to 30 minutes following a deep release. When getting up from the horizontal position, sit up slowly and have your patient sit at the side of the treatment table for 30 seconds or until dizziness has resolved. Patients on antihypertensive medication and patients prone to orthostatic hypotension should be carefully monitored. Measure their blood pressure before and after the myofascial treatment. Patients who have unstable angina should not receive myofascial treatment.

Specific muscles

The management of muscle pain in certain specific muscles have been elaborated in the below sections.

Deltoid

Location of Trigger Point
Anterior: three inches below the anterior margin of the acromion
Posterior: two inches distal to the posterior margin of the acromion

Referred Pain Pattern
Locally on the muscle; shoulder

Injury/ Cause of dysfunction
High velocity injuries related to sports; direct trauma to the muscle

Stretching Technique
Shoulder extension with elbow extension and neutral forearm
Horizontal adduction (from higher position) with elbow flexed (across body)

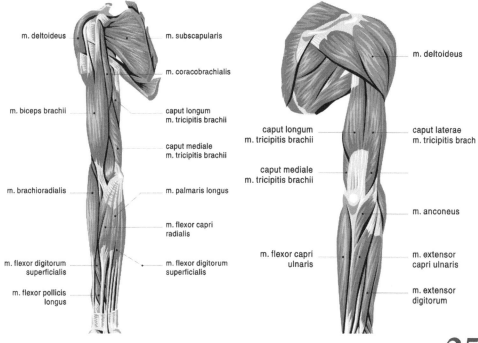

m. deltoideus
m. subscapularis
m. coracobrachialis
m. deltoideus
m. biceps brachii
caput longum
m. tricipitis brachii
m. biceps brachii
caput mediale
m. tricipitis brachii
caput longum
m. tricipitis brachii
caput laterae
m. tricipitis brach
caput mediale
m. tricipitis brachii
m. brachioradialis
m. palmaris longus
m. flexor capri
radialis
m. anconeus
m. flexor digitorum
superficialis
m. flexor digitorum
superficialis
m. flexor capri
ulnaris
m. extensor
capri ulnaris
m. flexor pollicis
longus
m. extensor
digitorum

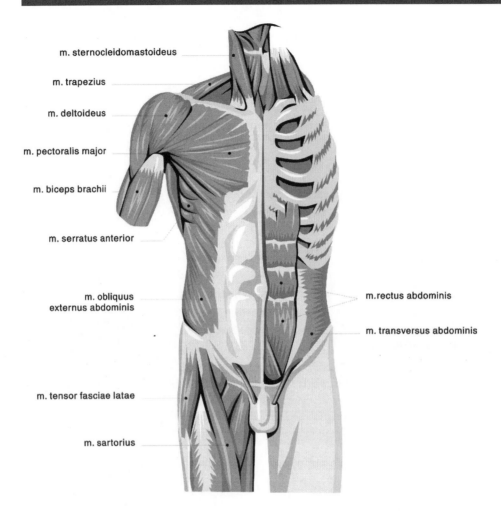

m. sternocleidomastoideus

m. trapezius

m. deltoideus

m. pectoralis major

m. biceps brachii

m. serratus anterior

m. obliquus externus abdominis

m.rectus abdominis

m. transversus abdominis

m. tensor fasciae latae

m. sartorius

Biceps Brachii

Location of Trigger Point
Two trigger points mid way, (pincer palpation) near insertion (flat palpation)

Referred Pain Pattern
Shoulder to the anterior elbow near the insertion of the muscle

Injury/ Cause of dysfunction
Sudden overstretching of the muscles, lifting heavy objects or following sports activities

Stretching Technique
Extension of the elbow with shoulder extended

Triceps

Location of Trigger Point
Belly of the muscle mid-arm (pincer)

Referred Pain Pattern
Posterior arm, medial or lateral epicondyle and fingers

Injury/ Cause of dysfunction
Sudden over stretching of the muscle, sports or lifting heavy objects.

Stretching Technique
Elbow flexion

Brachioradialis

Location of Trigger Point
Below the flexor crease and midway between the biceps tendon and lateral epicondyle

Referred Pain Pattern
Lateral epicondyle along the brachioradialis muscle and at web space

Injury/ Cause of dysfunction
Sports injury, wrist extension with pronated forearm

Stretching Technique
Elbow extension
Pronation
Wrist flexion
Ulnar deviation

Supinator

Location of Trigger Point
Radial and distal to the biceps tendon insertion

Referred Pain Pattern
Near biceps tendon and web space

Injury/ Cause of dysfunction
Sports, especially where supination is required

Stretching Technique
Elbow extension and pronation; wrist flexion ulnar deviation

Pronator Teres

Location of Trigger Point
Two inches distal to the midpoint of a line connecting the medial epicondyle and biceps tendon

Referred Pain Pattern
Radial side of wrist and anterior surface of the forearm

Injury/ Cause of dysfunction
Weight lifting, carrying babies (pronator syndrome)

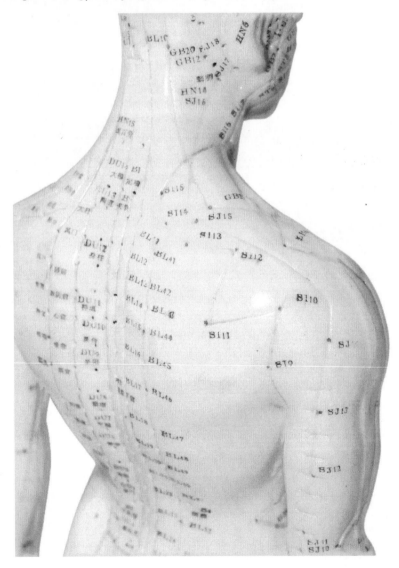

Stretching technique
Elbow extension and complete supination
Wrist extension

Flexor Carpi Ulnaris

Location of Trigger Point
Trigger finger (may contribute)

Referred Pain Pattern
Ulnar side of wrist (pisiform)

Injury/ Cause of dysfunction
Tight grip of large objects, prolonged grip

Stretching technique
Elbow extension
Supination
Wrist extension
Radial deviation

Flexor Carpi Radialis

Location of Trigger Point
3-4 inches below the midline connecting the medial epicondyle and biceps tendon

Referred Pain Pattern
Radial and anterior sides of the wrist near the wrist crease and carpal canal

Injury/ Cause of dysfunction
Repetitive finger and wrist motion

Stretching technique
Elbow extension
Supination
Wrist extension
Radial deviation

Extensor Carpi Radialis

Location of Trigger Point
Two inches distal to lateral epicondyle

Referred Pain Pattern
Wrist web space, lateral epicondyle and forearm

Injury/ Cause of dysfunction
Prolonged or repetitive extension of the wrist, typing, tennis, golf

Stretching Technique
Elbow extension
Pronation
Wrist flexion

Extensor Carpi Ulnaris

Location of Trigger Point
Midpoint of ulna; identified by flat palpation

Referred Pain Pattern
Ulnar and dorsal side of the wrist
Injury/ Cause of dysfunction
Prolonged or repetitive wrist extension, typing, playing tennis or golf

Stretching technique
Elbow extension
Pronation and wrist flexion

Extensor Digitorum

Location of Trigger Point
Four inches below lateral epicondyle

Referred Pain Pattern
Middle finger, forearm and lateral eipicondyle (radial tunnel)

Injury/ Cause of dysfunction
Repetitive finger movements commonly found in musicians, typists, dental hygienists

Stretching technique
Elbow extension
Pronation
Wrist flexion
Finger flexion

Extensor Indicis Proprius

Location of Trigger Point
Two inches proximal to the ulnar styloid in the interspace between ulna and radius

Referred Pain Pattern
Radial wrist and hand

Injury/ Cause of dysfunction
Direct trauma, repetitive motion such as typing or use of mouse, writing and playing musical instruments

Stretching technique
Wrist flexion
Index flexion

Abductor Pollicis Brevis

Location of Trigger Point
Midline of the first metacarpophalangeal joint of the thumb and the carpometacarpal joint

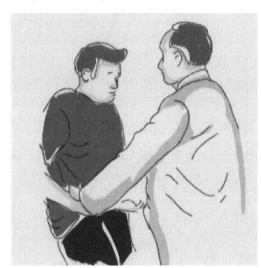

Referred Pain Pattern
Thenar eminence

Injury/ Cause of dysfunction
Handling, holding, grasping small objects, writing, painting; usually done by dentist, surgeons

Stretching technique
Extension of the thumb followed by adduction
Self stretch: May be involved in trigger thumb

Flexor Pollicis Brevis

Location of Trigger Point
Flat palpation; midline between the origin and insertion

Referred Pain Pattern
Volar and radial aspect of the thumb

Injury/ Cause of dysfunction
Prolonged small grasping, holding or handling, writing, painting, pinching hangers; commonly found on dental hygienists and jewelers

Stretching technique
Extension of the thumb

Adductor Pollicis

Location of Trigger Point
Web space, Pincer palpation
May be involved in trigger thumb

Referred Pain Pattern
Carpometacarpal joint area (radial and volar thumb)

Injury/ Cause of dysfunction
Handling and grasping small objects for prolonged periods of time

Stretching technique
Thumb abduction
Palmar or radial abduction
Home stretch of Adductor Pollicis
Use opposite hand to facilitate stretch

Levator Scapulae

Location of Trigger Point
Two inches below the angle of the neck and one inch medial

Referred Pain Pattern
Angle of the neck, along the vertebral border of scapula, posterior shoulder

Injury/ Cause of dysfunction
Overshortening of levator scapulae following ambulating with too long crutches or canes; carrying heavy bags supported by a belt over the shoulder

Stretching Technique
Neck flexion, side bending towards the opposite side, rotation to contralateral side

Upper trapezius

Location of Trigger Point
At the angle of neck

Referred Pain Pattern
Posterolateral aspect of the neck, behind the ear, temporal area up to the zygoma

Injury/ Cause of dysfunction
Active overshortening of the muscle due to actions such as stabilizing phone handset between neck and shoulder; carrying heavy bags supported by a belt over the shoulder

Stretching Technique
Neck flexion, side bending towards the opposite side, slight rotation to ipsilateral side

Muscle Energy Technique

Muscle energy techniques refers to a class of soft tissue osteopathic manipulation methods that incorporate precisely directed muscle contractions, designed to improve musculoskeletal function and reduce pain. It is aimed at restoring shortened structures to a normal resting length. Although variations exist, these techniques aim at toning inhibited musculature (Chaitow, 2006).

When a muscle is held in isometric contraction, its release is followed by a degree of relaxation not present prior to the contraction. When muscle fibers contract isometrically, approximation of the origin and insertion is prevented by an exactly equal counterforce. A marked release of increased tone will occur in the tissues. This contraction is maintained for a specific length of time (typically 7–10 seconds) after which relaxation is allowed. This allows a greater degree of pain-free stretch to take place in the shortened fibers. A new, but probably still limited, resting length is then achieved, and this is used as the starting position of the next isometric contraction. This phenomenon of post-isometric relaxation is used to sequentially stretch tight musculature in which myofascial trigger points are found. Once tight or shortened muscles have been relaxed and released, there is automatic toning of their previously inhibited antagonists. It is at this stage that rehabilitation can achieve results, as the individual learns better patterns of use and posture (Chaitow, 2006).

Postisometric relaxation

The post-isometric relaxation technique begins by placing the muscle in a stretched position. Then, an isometric contraction is exerted against minimal resistance. Relaxation and gentle stretch follow as the muscle releases. Postisometric relaxation is advised for stretching tissues housing active myofascial trigger points. The affected muscles are used in the isometric contraction; therefore, the shortened muscles subsequently relax via postisometric relaxation, allowing an easier stretch to be performed (Lewit & Simons, 1984).

The practitioner is attempting to push towards the barrier of restriction against the patient's precisely matched counter-effort. The therapist's and patient's forces are matched. Initial effort involves approximately 30% of patient's strength; an increase to no more than 40% on subsequent contractions may be appropriate. The duration of contraction is initially 7–10 seconds. Longer, stronger contractions may predispose towards onset of cramping. Therefore, a rest period of 5 seconds is necessary to ensure complete relaxation before commencing the stretch. On exhalation, the muscle is taken to its new restriction barrier and held in this position for at least 30 and up to 60 seconds. The patient should participate in assisting the stretch to retard the likelihood of a stretch reflex. This technique should be repeated three times (Lewit & Simons, 1984).

Postfacilitation stretch method

The shortened muscle is placed midrange position about halfway between a fully stretched and a fully relaxed state. Isometric contraction is performed for 5–10 seconds; while effort is resisted completely. On release, a rapid stretch without bounce is held for 10 seconds. The patient relaxes for 20 seconds. The process is repeated 3–5 times (Magnusson et al, 1996).

Reciprocal inhibition

Reciprocal inhibition refers to physiological response of the antagonists of a muscle that has been isometrically contracted. This has been reported to be an excellent method of treating the myofascial trigger phenomena where the muscle can achieve full resting length. Reciprocal Inhibition is indicated for stretching chronic or subacute restricted, fibrotic, contracted soft tissues (fascia, muscle), or tissues housing active myofascial trigger points. This approach is chosen if contracting the agonist is contraindicated because of pain. The starting point is short of the

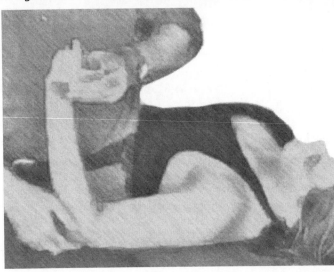

resistance barrier. The antagonists to the affected muscles are used in the isometric contraction; therefore, the shortened muscles subsequently relax via reciprocal inhibition, allowing an easier stretch to be performed. The patient is attempting to push towards the barrier of restriction, against the practitioner's precisely matched counter-effort. The practitioner's and patient's forces are matched. Initial effort involves approximately 30% of patient's strength. The duration of contraction is initially 7–10 seconds, increasing to up to 15 seconds in subsequent contractions. There should be a rest period of 5 seconds to ensure complete relaxation before commencing the stretch. On exhalation, the muscle is taken to its new restriction barrier and held in this position for at least 30 seconds. The patient should participate in assisting in the stretch to prevent the stretch reflex. This procedure should be repeated three times or until no further gain in range of motion is possible.

Muscle Energy concepts

According to Mitchell (1991), individuals who have problems that respond well to muscle energy techniques often give a history of a previous injury. These individuals will often relate their chronic problems to some injury in the past. This injury is sometimes a focal point in their minds and their life seems to be affected around this injury.

Dr. Mitchell recommends the following protocol:

1. Identify the dysfunction.

2. Position the part to be treated in a loose pack position. This position is sometimes referred to as ease/bind position.

3. The above position is found by positioning the part in all three planes of motion and backing off from the barrier when it is located.

4. The clinician now instructs the patient to make a light contraction in that direction.

5. The clinician resists the very light contraction.

6. When the correct level of contraction is reached, the clinician instructs the patient to hold the contraction steady at this level.

7. At this point, the clinician begins a count of 6 seconds. This appears to be the amount of time needed to reset the gamma gain in the muscle. (Gamma gain appears to represent the amount of muscular activity occurring in the muscular tissue holding the joint in a dysfunctional position.)

8. At the end of 6 seconds, the clinician instructs the patient to relax the contraction. The muscles controlling the joint now have a different gamma gain, and the neutral position of the joint will now be different.

9. The clinician now repositions the joint utilizing the steps outlined in number 3 above.

10. The clinician now repeats steps 4 through 8 outlined above.

11. At the end of the second contraction, the gamma gain will again be altered so a new position can be obtained. The reduction in gamma gain will be greatest following this second contraction.

12. At the end of the third contraction, the muscles of the joint should be stretched out. This seems to greatly increase the effectiveness of the treatment.

13. If the range of motion of the joint is now acceptable, the treatment is now considered complete.

Effect of Breathing

Alterations in breathing techniques can also lead to microtrauma or muscle fatigue over a period of time. Activity of phrenic motoneurons contributes to posture and respiration (Hodges, 2001). Frank hyperventilation may cause alkalization caused by breathing. These respiratory muscles can become prone to fatigue, dysfunction, and trigger point evolution (Norris, 1999).

Positional Release Technique

The concept of positional release revolves around releasing undesirable stress being experienced by the muscles. Positional release technique involves the placement of soft tissues or joints into positions of ease to encourage self-regulating influences to operate more efficiently, resulting in greater range of motion and reduced pain (Chaitow, 2007).

There are different positional release methods wherein the modalities such as stretching, massaging, mobilization, or manipulation may be used to achieve the desired results. Osteopathic medicine has contributed three major positional release techniques that include strain-counterstrain, functional technique, and facilitated positional release (Chaitow, 2009).

Strain-Counterstrain Technique (SCS)

Strain-counterstrain is a progressive manual therapy technique specifically addressing dysfunctional muscles. Passively shortening the over stimulated muscle and lengthening of the antagonist will result in a decrease in firing of the afferent neuron. In return, a decrease in excitation of the gamma neuron will result in decreased activity in the extrafusal and intrafusal muscle fibers (Rodriguez-Blanco et al, 2006).

Strain-Counterstrain Technique works through the discovery of tender points. A tender point can be classified as a tense, tender, edematous muscle and fascial tissue 1 cm in diameter, with no referral pattern. Dr. Lawrence Jones has

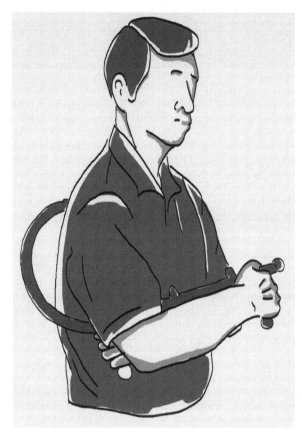

discovered close to 200 tender points that correlate with a specific dysfunction (Rodriguez-Blanco et al, 2006).

Tender points are not just subjective. The clinician can feel changes in tissue tension. The patient should be positioned in a posture of maximum relaxation. While treatments are done once a week to each tender point found, about six points maximum are done per session. This allows a period of adjustment and may in turn shut off other tender points. Patient education is also very important. For example, a patient with back pain may have a tender point in the abdomen at the area of the iliacus. Explain to the patient the origin and insertion of this muscle and how it may be causing low back pain. The patient can place a pillow under the buttocks, cross the legs at the ankles and flex the legs towards the stomach. With a slight adjustment in bending to the side opposite of tenderness, the tender point will be turned off. After a 90-second hold and a slow movement back to neutral, the pain will have decreased by 70% (Rodriguez-Blanco et al, 2006).

In strain-counterstrain methodology, a palpated sensitive point is used as a monitor to guide the tissues towards ease, via feedback from the patient. As the reported pain level reduces (from a starting point of 10/10 to 3/10 or less), the tissues being palpated are felt to become slacker and less tense. The ease position is then held for 90 seconds or so, before being gently released (Rodriguez-Blanco et al, 2006).

The strain-counterstrain technique works to inhibit hyperactivity of the spasm reflex, allowing the muscle to relax by improving oxygenation and eliminating pain. Strain-counterstrain involves maintaining pressure on the monitored tender point, or periodically probing it, as a position is achieved in which there is no additional pain in the area and the pain point has reduced by at least 70% (Rodriguez-Blanco et al, 2006).

There are several settings where the strain-counterstrain techniques are indicated. These include reduction of stiffness in pre- and post-operative patients, muscle spasm cases where other direct methods may not be tolerated, acute and multiple strains, such as whiplash injuries, and management of chronic soft tissue dysfunction (Rodriguez-Blanco et al, 2006).

Three important pointers in performing strain-counterstrain technique include: (a) locate and palpate the appropriate tender point; (b) use minimal force; (c) achieve a position of maximum ease or comfort where no additional pain is produced anywhere else in the body.

Application Guidelines

Find a pain point, which is usually in shortened muscles. (For example, if you find it painful to move in a particular direction, say turning your head to the left, then there may be shortness in the muscles that turn your head to the right.)

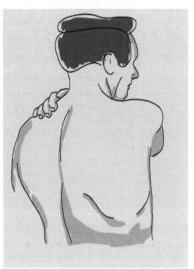

Press on the point of tenderness hard enough to score '10'.

Move your body, or the part of the body, around slowly until the pain is reduced to a '3', causing no additional pain or new pain anywhere else.

Stay in that position of 'ease' for 1 minute. Slowly return to neutral.

Care should be taken while treating patients with malignancy, aneurysm, and acute inflammatory conditions. Strain-counterstrain is contraindicated in skin conditions that restrict the application of pressure and following recent major trauma or surgery. Increase in pain during the procedure contraindicates further progression. Caution should also be taken while placing the neck in extension.

Integrated Neuromuscular Inhibition Technique

The integrated neuromuscular inhibition technique is based on the hypothesis that combining the methods of direct inhibition (through progressive pressure or through ischemic compression), strain-counterstrain, and muscle

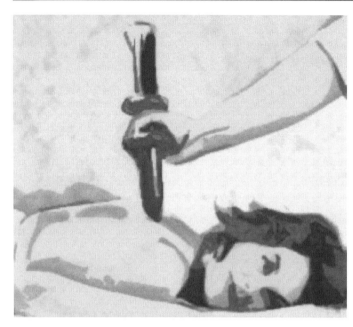

energy technique can help target the tissues in which the trigger point is housed so that when stretching is introduced, the fibrotic musculature is able to regain its normal resting length (Chaitow, 2009).

Application Guidelines

Locate the trigger point by means of 'STAR' palpation. Apply ischemic compression or progressive pressure until a significant release is noted in the palpated tissues. Positionally release trigger point tissues using the strain-counterstrain technique. Pressure is applied and the patient is asked to ascribe this a value of '10', and then tissues are repositioned (fine-tuned) until the patient reports a score of '3' or less. Apply local stretch to the tissues housing the trigger point in the direction of the muscle fibers. Then, the whole muscle is then contracted isometrically. This is followed by a stretch of the whole muscle as described in the muscle energy technique (Chaitow, 2009).

Instrument Assisted Myofascial Release

While touch provides the feedback of temperature, moisture, contours, and communication that cannot be duplicated by instrumentation, the use of instruments can considerably improve skills by magnifying the sensation of

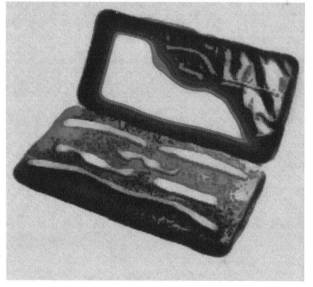

touch, detect involved areas of the kinetic chain more efficiently, reach areas of increased depth, conserve the therapist's joints, and dramatically improve the treatment outcomes (Loghmani & Warden, 2009).

The use of instruments for therapy is an ancient practice. To penetrate deep areas that are difficult to reach with the hands, T-bars that were made of wood and had rubber tips have been used for centuries. Ancient East Asian methods, like Gua Sha, make use of any smooth edge, such as buffalo horn or even the metal lid from a jar. The concept of Gua sha is based on the explanation that promoting blood production and improving the dissemination of fluids improves healing. This effect can be brought about by scraping the skin and attracting blood from the tissue or causing small petechiae or ecchymotic patches. 37 In recent times, lucite, acrylic, ceramics, and stainless steel instruments are widely used (Nielsen, 2000).

Effects of manual loading on soft tissue

Instrumentation on the soft tissue brings about the stimulation of fibroblasts and their synthesis of proteoglycan and collagen. The goal of healing in conditions such as tendinosis is to enhance the proliferative invasion of vascular elements and fibroblasts, followed by collagen deposition and ultimate maturation. In fact, application of mechanical load literally creates new tissue and helps it mature, when followed by specific stretching and strengthening. It has been specified that dynamic strain aids in fibroblast stimulation and in the organization of extracellular matrix of connective tissues. Several authors have noted the benefits of use of instruments in myofascial therapy. Davidson, et al. (1997) demonstrated that tendon healing occurred by the activation of fibroblasts following the use of augmented soft-tissue mobilization (augmented soft tissue mobilization-instrument-assisted).

Gehlsen, et al. (1999) found that the use of instruments increased the number and size of fibroblasts. They found that heavy pressure promoted the healing process to a greater degree than light or moderate pressure.

It is noted that friction massage can increase blood circulation and fibroblastic proliferation, wherein friction should be applied for 20 minutes or more. It has been believed that controlled microtrauma caused by instrumentation results in microvascular trauma and capillary hemorrhage, thereby creating a localized inflammatory response that can stimulate the body's healing cascade and the immune or reparative system. Prentice states that tendon healing is facilitated by accelerating the inflammatory process (Hammer, 2004).

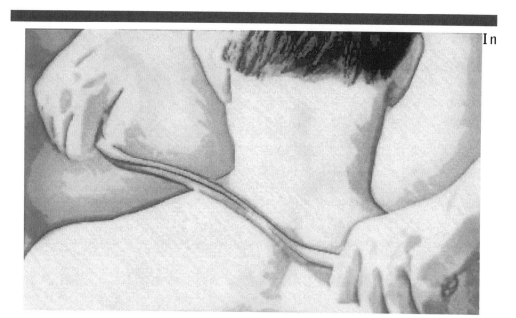

addition to the benefits of enhanced mechanical load, the sensation resulting from palpation of soft-tissue adhesions with the use of instruments can be magnified to a great extent. Clinicians who use these techniques report that they can feel blockages more precisely, both in terms of location and barrier direction. Another major benefit of the use of instrumentation is the preservation of the joints of the practitioner.

Benefits of Cross fiber massage

Cross-fiber massage is a method for accelerating and/or augmenting capsular and extracapsular ligament healing in case of ligament injuries. The process of cross-fiber massage involves the application of specifically directed forces in a direction transverse to the underlying collagen substructure with an intention of inducing physiological and structural tissue changes.

The use of rigid instruments for delivering cross-fiber massage has been referred to as the instrument-assisted cross-fiber massage technique. The technique ensures faster healing assisted by tissue remodeling. Results of some clinical pilot studies performed to evaluate the benefits of instrument assisted cross fiber massage also suggest that this technique reduced symptoms in individuals with conditions such as carpal tunnel syndrome, patellar tendinopathy, and chronic ankle pain (Burke et al, 2007).

The study that evaluated the use of instrument assisted cross fiber massage in treating acute capsular and extracapsular ligament injury has suggested that instrument assisted cross fiber massage may accelerate early tissue-level healing in acute capsular and extracapsular ligament injuries but it has minimal to no effect in terms of augmenting the overall outcome of the ligament-healing process. It may facilitate earlier return of ligament tissue-level biomechanical properties, enabling quicker return to function with less susceptibility to reinjury (Nirschl & Ashman, 2003).

Graston Technique

The Graston Technique makes use of six specially designed stainless steel instruments with beveled edges for the purpose of diagnosis and treatment. The Graston technique is based on the scientific literature describing the effects of manual loading on soft tissue. One of the most important findings regarding the effect of instrumentation on soft tissue is the stimulation of fibroblasts and their synthesis of proteoglycan and collagen (Falvey, 2000).

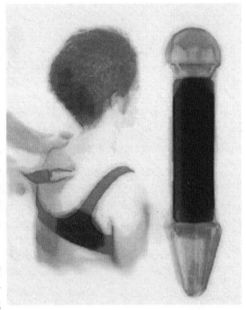

The Graston technique also referred to as Graston Instrument-Assisted Soft Tissue Mobilization uses a specialized form of massage to breakdown scar tissues and promotes faster healing. The therapist reintroduces a controlled amount of microtrauma using the cross-friction massage technique. This involves brushing or rubbing against the grain of the scar tissue with the instruments. There are several conditions wherein the Graston Instrument-Assisted Soft Tissue Mobilization has been noted to be beneficial. Some of the conditions for which this therapy is widely used include carpal tunnel syndrome, plantar fasciitis, cervical sprain/strain, lumbar sprain/strain, Achilles tendinitis, patellofemoral disorders, rotator cuff tendinitis, lateral epicondylitis, and medial epicondylitis (Falvey, 2000).

The instruments act as an extension of the provider's hands. A typical session consists of about eight to ten sessions conducted two days apart over four to five weeks wherein marked improvements can be expected between the fourth and the sixth visits. This technique is generally not used alone and is considered to be a vital part of therapy.

Augmented Soft Tissue Mobilization (ASTYM)

Augmented soft tissue mobilization is a modification of traditional soft tissue mobilization technique wherein certain specifically designed solid instruments are used to perform the mobilization. These instruments, rather than the hands and fingers of the therapist, are used to provide the contact mobilization force in the treatment of conditions.

The results of the study by Davidson et al. (1997) not only demonstrated improved limb function following augmented soft tissue mobilization treatment, but also suggested that augmented soft tissue mobilization may facilitate tendon healing by recruiting and activating fibroblasts.

The ASTYM System is a form of augmented soft tissue mobilization (augmented soft tissue mobilization) which allows the therapist to stimulate the body's own capacity for healing in patients suffering from soft tissue degeneration or fibrosis and chronic inflammation. This non-invasive treatment is performed to initiate the healing process necessary for tissue remodeling.

Adhesions and inappropriate fibrosis can occur within soft tissue as a result of processes such as trauma, surgery, immobilization, or repetitive strain. The ASTYM System stimulates the breakdown of these dysfunctional tissues, thereby allowing functional restoration to occur. Controlled microtraumas can initiate a local inflammatory response that can lead to the resorption of inappropriate fibrosis or excessive scar tissue in the affected areas. In chronic tendonopathies, delivering multiple doses of controlled microtrauma can stimulate the regeneration of the affected tendons. Existing collagen can be remodeled and formation of new collagen can be brought about by program specific functional activities and stretching.

Some of the clinical diagnoses that have responded well to ASTYM therapy include lateral epicondylitis, carpal tunnel syndrome, DeQuervain's tenosynovitis, trigger finger, joint contractures, iliotibial band syndrome, patellar tendinitis, shin splints, chronic ankle sprains, Achilles tendinitis, and plantar fascit is (Wilson et al, 2000).

This section describes the outcomes of several studies which evaluated the benefits of myofascial treatment programs. Here, the outcomes of the studies are discussed with its implications on current practice methods.

Eight-week calf myofascial treatment programs

Wu et al. (2009) investigated the influence of the chronic calf muscle tightness caused by myofascial pain syndrome. Myofascial pain syndrome is a common clinical problem of muscle pain caused by myofascial trigger points. The chronic muscle tightness caused by myofascial pain syndrome is a factor influencing the joint motion.

The study involved the use of an eight-week calf myofascial treatment program that included several manual techniques such as deep myofascial release, deep friction massage, and proprioceptive neuromuscular facilitation, stretching and home program. At the end of the therapy, significant improvements in the ankle-dorsiflexion range of motion of the affected leg were noted. Moderate improvement in pain during resting and after work was also recorded. The authors noted that the myofascial treatments improved the clinical symptoms and kinetics of gait.

Home Program of Ischemic Pressure and Sustained Stretch for Myofascial Trigger Points

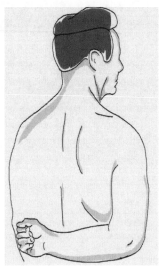

The effectiveness of a home program of ischemic pressure followed by sustained stretching for the treatment of myofascial trigger points in adults with one or more myofascial trigger points in the neck or upper back was evaluated by Hanten et al (2000). The study involved a five-day home program of ischemic pressure followed by general sustained stretching of the neck and upper back musculature for the experimental group or active range of motion for the control group. The measurements were based on scoring criteria such as pressure pain threshold and the visual analog scale.

The results of the study demonstrated the effectiveness of ischemic pressure followed by sustained stretching in reducing myofascial trigger points sensitivity as measured with a pressure algometer and pain intensity scored with a visual analogue scale. Stretching of the affected muscle is believed to be an integral part of myofascial trigger point therapy. The stretching techniques such as post-isometric relaxation technique have been effective in reducing myofascial trigger points' sensitivity and pain intensity. The authors concluded that clinicians can manage neck and upper back pain associated with myofascial trigger points through a home program of ischemic pressure and sustained stretching with periodic monitoring by a therapist.55 Therefore, the effectiveness of stretching in the release of myofascial trigger points is also noted in home therapy programs.

Ease of technique reproducibility

The ease of the learning and identifying strain-counterstrain points was evaluated by Tatom and Laman (1999) who performed a study to determine the intertester reliability of identifying strain and counterstrain points between a certified instructor of the Jones Institute and clinicians with first-time didactic instructions of the technique. Following a brief introduction to the concepts involved in counterstrain, a demonstration and instruction were given on manual techniques for discovering the first six anterior thoracic tender points on the sternum. The trained individuals were supposed to demonstrate the learned technique. It was noted that all the trained individuals performed successfully in this study. The results of this pilot study demonstrated that the technique could easily be reproduced accurately and highlights the ease of learning these procedures.

Myofascial pain and fibromyalgia: Thorough history necessary

Chronic muscle pain (myalgia) is a common problem that is a difficult problem for the clinician who is interested in the management of pain. A thorough analysis and proper selection of the treatment plan is highly necessary to obtain optimal results. While myofascial trigger point release is beneficial, identifying the underlying cause and managing it appropriately is also equally important.

In many instances, patients suffering from myalgia can have numerous co-morbid conditions that may perpetuate the pain. Some of these causes of chronic myalgia can include structural causes such as scoliosis, localized joint hypomobility, and generalized or localized joint laxity. Metabolic factors include depleted tissue iron stores, hypothyroidism, and Vitamin D deficiency.

These conditions may interfere with the recovery or treatment process; therefore, identification of such underlying conditions should be undertaken in all patients. In some instances, physical examination may reveal an obvious structural abnormality, while in others; a detailed history and laboratory examination may be required to identify the root cause of the problem. The presence of multiple co-morbidities, such as having a combination of a structural imbalance and a medical condition, is not uncommon. In several instances, correction of an underlying cause of myalgia is all that is needed to resolve the condition. Therefore, proper diagnosis and treatment can eliminate pain in numerous individuals suffering from chronic myalgia.

Effect of myofascial release on an adult with idiopathic scoliosis

Idiopathic scoliosis is classified as a patient having at least a 10° lateral curve of the spine for which a recognizable cause is unknown. Rotational deformities can lead to abnormal or reduced respiratory function, which may lead to serious respiratory impairments, pain, and a decrease in the patient's quality of life (Upadhyay et al, 1995).

The study by LeBauer et al. (2008) measured the effects of myofascial release as a manual therapy technique in the treatment of idiopathic scoliosis. Six weeks of myofascial release treatment consisting of two sessions each week for sixty minutes were provided. Pain, pulmonary function, and quality of life were measured. Range of motion measurements were taken for trunk flexion, extension, and rotation. Following six weeks of treatment, improvements in thoracolumbar rotation and posture were noted. Pain levels, quality of life measures, and pulmonary function improved significantly. The results of this study suggest further investigation is needed using myofascial release as an effective manual therapy treatment for idiopathic scoliosis.

Changes in active mouth opening following a single treatment of latent myofascial trigger points in the masseter muscle involving post-isometric relaxation or strain-counterstrain

Ninety subjects (42 men, mean age 25 years) with a latent myofascial trigger points in the masseter muscle were selected. Myofascial trigger points were identified using the Simons, Travell and Simons criteria. The immediate effect on active mouth opening following a single treatment with either post-isometric relaxation or strain-counterstrain technique was studied (Rodriguez et al, 2006).

Subjects were randomly assigned to one of three groups. The first group received post-isometric relaxation, the second group received strain-counterstrain, and the third group functioned as the control group that received no treatment. Treatment by post-isometric relaxation began with passive opening of the mouth followed by isometric contraction. This is repeated three times. Strain-counterstrain by the therapist involved applying pressure to the masseter myofascial trigger point by pincer palpation until the subject felt pain. Then, the subject was passively positioned into a position of ease that reduced the palpable tension and pain by around 75%, which was ipsilateral side flexion of the cervical spine and a slight mouth opening [5–8 mm]. Blinded evaluations of mouth opening before treatment, and five minutes post-treatment found an increase of 2.0 mm after post-isometric relaxation, 0.2 mm after strain-counterstrain, [p < 0.001], and 0.1 mm for the control group. Only the group receiving post-isometric relaxation showed a significant improvement in active mouth opening (Rodriguez et al, 2006).

Sympathetic facilitation of hyperalgesia evoked from myofascial tender and trigger points in patients with unilateral shoulder pain

Twenty-one female subjects with an active myofascial trigger point in one of the infraspinatus muscles causing chronic unilateral shoulder pain were included in this study. A tender point in the contralateral infraspinatus muscle was identified. A point in the right tibialis anterior muscle was used as a control point. Subjects rated their resting pain on a visual analog scale before any measurements were taken. The researchers determined the pressure pain threshold using an algometer during normal respiration and during induced elevated intrathoracic pressure, which is described as a maneuver that increases the sympathetic outflow to the skeletal muscle when holding one's breath with the glottis closed. With this maneuver, it is possible to determine the effect of increased sympathetic outflow on the mechanical sensitivity of myofascial trigger points (Ge et al, 2006).

In the second phase of the study, the pressure pain threshold and the pressure threshold for eliciting referred pain were determined in eleven subjects. The local pain and referred pain intensities were measured during normal respiration and during induced elevated intrathoracic pressure while applying 1.5x pressure to elicit referred pain. After all measures were completed, a local twitch response was elicited in the active myofascial trigger points using an acupuncture needle. The authors concluded that increasing sympathetic outflow to the muscle decreases pressure pain threshold, myofascial trigger points, and increased local and referred pain intensities at both tender and trigger points (Ge et al, 2006).

Proximal hamstring rupture, restoration of function without surgical intervention

A 26-year old female tennis player and runner suffered a hyperextension injury of her left knee while water skiing, which resulted in a proximal rupture of the biceps femoris, semimembranosus, and semitendinosus. Although medical consensus dictates that surgical repair is the best treatment for hamstrings ruptures, the patient declined surgical intervention and opted for physical therapy instead. After the first course of physical therapy, which included hydrotherapy, electrotherapy, and exercise, she had regained a 60% improvement in power as assessed isokinetically, but she was not able to return to athletic activities, especially running. She was referred to another physical therapist, who evaluated her for the presence of myofascial trigger points. At that point, she was already 19 months post-injury. Her running capacity was limited to only 4–5 minutes with increased pain after 3–4 days (Grieve, 2006).

The patient presented with multiple myofascial trigger points in the left hamstrings and gastrocnemius. The objectives of physical therapy were to restore her pre-injury athletic ability, reduce the sensitivity of the myofascial trigger points, and increase the power of the hamstrings. During the first treatment session, the physical therapist used progressive pressure release and passive stretching, which resulted in an immediate increase in ankle dorsiflexion and hamstrings strength (Grieve, 2006).

A week later, the patient reported being able to dance an entire night. There was only one sensitive myofascial trigger point left. After the third physical therapy session, she was able to run six minutes daily without any post-activity pain. She still had one myofascial trigger point in the semimembranosus muscle. She had reached her treatment goals by the fourth session. Long-term follow up at three and six months revealed no further pain and dysfunction (Grieve, 2006).

Trigger points in tension-type headache

Twenty patients with chronic tension-type headache and twenty matched controls without headache were examined for active and latent myofascial trigger points. A blinded assessor made photographic measures of forward head posture and each subject kept a headache diary for four weeks. Sixty-five percent of the patients had active myofascial trigger points and thirty-five percent of them had latent myofascial trigger points in the suboccipital muscles. The difference in active myofascial trigger points was statistically significant (P< 0.05). Forward head posture was greater in patients than in controls, both when sitting and standing, P<0.01. The authors concluded that the frequency and duration of chronic tension-type headache and the degree of forward head posture correlated positively with the presence of active suboccipital myofascial trigger points (Nixon & Andrews, 1996).

Active fascial contractility: Fascia can influence musculoskeletal dynamics

Dense connective tissue sheets, commonly known as fascia, play an important role as force transmitters in human posture and movement regulation. Fascia is usually seen as having a passive role, transmitting mechanical tension which is generated by muscle activity or external forces. However, there is some evidence to suggest that fascia may be able to actively contract in a smooth muscle-like manner and consequently influence musculoskeletal dynamics (Schleip, 2005).

General support for this hypothesis came with the discovery of contractile cells in fascia. Evidence to support this hypothesis is offered by in vitro studies with the biomechanical demonstration of an autonomous contraction of the human lumbar fascia, and the pharmacological induction of temporary contractions in normal fascia from rats. If verified by future research, the existence of an active fascial contractility could have interesting implications for the understanding of musculoskeletal pathologies. It may also offer new insights on myofascial trigger point release therapies or trigger point acupuncture. Further research to test this hypothesis is suggested (Schleip, 2005).

Conclusion

The body has a natural healing capacity that needs to be harnessed to treat myofascial conditions. Hippocrates urged his students to facilitate natural healing. The popularity of myofascial therapy is increasing and has been gaining medical acceptance. Therapists from diverse educational backgrounds have been utilizing myofascial therapeutic and diagnostic methods for centuries. While the critics of myofascial therapy tend to increase the controversy related to this type of therapy, the gap between the consumers and critics of this therapy will eventually be bridged by the instincts common to both groups.

A wide number of analytic studies are being conducted to evaluate the safety and efficacy of the different myofascial trigger point release techniques. Additionally, studies are also being conducted to define different conditions and situations where myofascial release techniques may be beneficial. The concepts of myofascial release that were first discussed in the 19th century continue to evolve. The industrial revolution and the modern inventions in the fields of science and technology have helped this continuous process with the development of several different instruments. This has aided the practitioner in diagnosis and treatment of these musculoskeletal conditions (Leadbetter, 1992 and Lewit, 1999).

Research indicates that myofascial release provides pain relief, improved posture, and improved quality of life. The only limitation noted with the use of myofascial release is the knowledge and skill required by the individual practitioner. Nevertheless, the revolution in the field of information technology has increased the access to knowledge and also opened up newer methods of developing the required skills. With proper dedication and support from the scientific community, myofascial release therapy is all set to revolutionize the field of medicine.

Beaulieu, J. (1981). Developing a stretching program. Physician and Sports Medicine, 9(11), 59–69.

Burke, J., Buchberger, D. J., Carey-Loghmani, M. T., Dougherty, P. E., Greco, D. S., & Dishman, J. D. (2007). A pilot study comparing two manual therapy interventions for carpal tunnel syndrome. Journal of manipulative and physiological therapeutics, 30(1), 50–61. doi: 10.1016/j.jmpt.2006.11.014

Chaitow, L. (2006). Muscle energy techniques: Advanced soft tissue techniques (3rd ed.). Philadelphia : Elsevier Health Sciences.

Chaitow, L. (Ed.). (2007). Positional release techniques (3rd ed.). Edinburgh: Churchill Livingstone.

Chaitow, L. (2009). Ligaments and positional release techniques. Journal of Bodywork and Movement Therapies, 13(2), 115–116. Retrieved from http://www.leonchaitow.com/PDFs/LigamentsPositionalRelease.pdf

Cyriax, J. (1984). Textbook of orthopaedic medicine: Treatment by manipulation, massage and injection (Wol. 2, 11th ed.). London, Bailliere Tindall.

Davidson, C. J., Ganion, L. R., Gehlsen, G. M., Verhoestra B., Roepke J. E. , Sevier T.L. (1997). Rat tendon morphologic and functional changes resulting from soft tissue mobilization. Medicine and science in sports and exercise, 29(3),313–319.

DiGiovanna, E., Stanley, S., & Dowling, D. J. (2005). Myofascial (soft tissue) techniques: An osteopathic approach to diagnosis and treatment (3rd ed.). Philadelphia: Lippincott Williams & Wilkins.

East Tenessee State Unitverity. (2001). Histology of muscle. Retrieved from http://faculty.etsu.edu/forsman/Histologyofmuscleforweb.htm

Eastwood, M., McGrouther, D.A., Brown, R.A. (1998). Fibroblast responses to mechanical forces. Proceedings of the Institution of Mechanical Engineers. Part H, Journal of engineering in medicine, 212(2), 85-92.

Evjenth, O., & Hamberg, J. (1984). Muscle stretching in manual therapy. Sweden: Alfta.

Falvey, M. (2000). Repetitive stress injuries: Fighting back with the Graston technique. Claims, 4(5), 38–46.

51

Fernández-de-las-Peñas, C., Alonso-Blanco, C., Cuadrado, M. L., Gerwin, R. D., & Pareja, J. A. (2006). Trigger points in the suboccipital muscles and forward head posture in tension- type headache. Headache, 46(3), 454–460. doi: 10.1111/j.1526-4610.2006.00288.x

Fleckenstein, D. J. (2009). Trigger points and classical acupuncture points: Part 3; Relationships of myofascial referred pain patterns to acupuncture meridians. Deutsche Zeitschrift für Akupunktur, 52(1), 9–14.

Galantino, M. L., Bzdewka, T. M., Eissler-Russo, J. L., Holbrook, M. L., Mogck, E.P., Geigle, P.,

Farrar, J.T. (2004). The impact of modified hatha yoga on chronic low back pain: A pilot study. Alternative Therapies in Health and Medicine, 10(2), 56–59.

Ge, H. Y., Fernández-de-las-Peñas, C., & Arendt-Nielsen, L. (2006). Sympathetic facilitation of hyperalgesia evoked from myofascial tender and trigger points in patients with unilateral shoulder pain. Clinical Neurophysiology, 117(7), 1545–1550. doi: 10.1016/j.clinph.2006.03.026

Gehlsen, G. M., Ganion, L. R., & Helfst, R. (1999). Fibroblast responses to variation in soft tissue mobilization pressure. Medicine and science in sports and exercise, 31(4), 531–535.

Gerwin, R. D. (2005). A review of myofascial pain and fibromyalgia: Factors that promote their persistence. Acupuncture In Medicine, 23(3), 121–134. Retrieved from http://aim.bmj.com/content/23/3/121.long

Grieve, G. (1986). Modern manual therapy. London: Churchill Livingstone.

Grieve, R. (2006). Proximal hamstring rupture, restoration of function without surgical intervention: A case study on myofascial trigger point pressure release. Journal of Bodywork & Movement Therapies, 10(2), 99–104. doi: 10.1016/j.jbmt.2005.08.003

Gross, M. T. (1992). Acute and Chronic Tendon Injuries: Factors Affecting the Healing Response and Treatment. Journal of Orthopaedic & Sports Physical Therapy, 16(6), 248–261.

Hammer, W. (2004). Instrument-assisted soft-tissue mobilization: A scientific and clinical perspective. Dynamic Chiropractic, 22(11). 1–4. Retrieved from http://www.grastontechnique.com/file/sites%7C*%7C86%7C*%7C2004_ InstrumentAssistedSoftTissueMobilization_ ScientificandClinicalPerspective_Hammer_DynamicChiropractic_2004.pdf. pdf

Han, S. C., & Harrison, P. (1997). Myofascial pain syndrome and trigger-point management Regional Anesthesia and Pain Medicine, 22(1), 89–101.

Hanten, W. P, Olson, S. L., Butts, N. L., & Nowicki, A. L. (2000). Effectiveness of a home program of ischemic pressure followed by sustained stretch for treatment of myofascial trigger points. Physical Therapy, 80(10), 997–1003. Retrieved from http://ptjournal.apta.org/content/80/10/997.full

Hodges, P. (2001). Postural activity of the diaphragm is reduced in humans when respiratory demand increases. The Journal of Physiology, 537(3), 999–1008. doi: 10.1111/j.1469-7793.2001.00999.x

Imamura, S. T., Fischer, A. A., Imamura, M., Teixeira M. J., Lin, T. Y., Kaziyama H.S., et al. (1997). Pain management using myofascial approach when other treatment failed. Physical Medicine & Rehabilitation Clinics of North America, 8(1), 179–96.

Jacobs, A., & Walls, W. (1997). Anatomy. In R. Ward (Ed.), Foundations of osteopathic medicine (pp. 15–58). Baltimore: Willliams and Wilkins.

Janda, V. (1993). Presentation to physical medicine research foundation Montreal Oct 9-11.

Kostopoulos, D., & Rizopoulos, K. (2001). The manual of trigger point and myofascial therapy. NY: Slack Incorporated.

Lavelle, E., Lavelle, W., & Smith, H. (2007). Myofascial trigger points. Medical Clinics of North America, 91(2), 229–239.

LeBauer, A., Brtalik, R., & Stowe, K. (2008). The effect of myofascial release (MFR) on an adult with idiopathic scoliosis. Journal of Bodywork and Movement Therapies, 12(4), 356–363. doi: 10.1016/j.jbmt.2008.03.008

Leadbetter, W. B. (1992). Cell-matrix response in tendon injury. Clinics in sports medicine, 11(3), 533– 577.

Lewit, K. (1999). Manipulation in rehabilitation of the locomotor system (3rd ed.) London: Butterworths.

Lewit, K., & Simons, D. G. (1984). Myofascial pain: Relief by post-isometric relaxation. Archives of physical medicine and rehabilitation, 65(8), 452–6.

Loghmani, M. T., & Warden, S. J. (2009). Instrument-assisted cross-fiber massage accelerates knee ligament healing. The Journal of orthopaedic and sports physical therapy, 39(7), 506–514. doi: 10.2519/jospt.2009.2997

Lundon, K. (2003). Orthopedic rehabilitation science: Principles for clinical management of nonmineralized connective tissue. St Louis: Elsevier Science.

Magnusson, S. P., Simonsen, E. B., Aagaard, P., Dyhre-Poulsen, P., McHugh, M., Kjaer, M., (1996). Mechanical and physiological responses to stretching with and without pre-isometric contraction in human skeletal muscle. Archives of Physical Medicine and Rehabilitation, 77(2), 373–377. doi: 10.1016/ S0003-9993(96)90087-8

Mattes, A. (1995). Flexibility: Active and assisted stretching. Sarasota: Mattes.

McAtee, R., & Charland, J. (1999). Facilitated stretching (2nd ed.). Champaign, IL: Human Kinetics.

Melham, T. J., Sevier, T. L., Malnofski, M. J., Wilson, J. K., & Helfst, R. H. (1998). Chronic ankle pain and fibrosis successfully treated with a new noninvasive augmented soft tissue mobilization technique (ASTM): a case report. Medicine and science in sports and exercise, 30(6), 801–804.

Melzack, R., & Wall, P. (1988). The challenge of pain. New York: Penguin.

Mitchell, F. L., & Mitchell, P. K. G. (1995). The muscle energy manual. City: MET Press.

Nielsen, A. (2000). Gua Sha: A traditional technique for modern practice. Edinburgh: Churchill Livingstone.

Nirschl, R. P., & Ashman, E. S. (2003). Elbow tendinopathy: tennis elbow. Clinics in sports medicine, 22(4), 813–836.

Nixon, P., & Andrews, J. (1996). A study of anaerobic threshold in chronic fatigue syndrome (CFS). Biological Psychology, 43(3), 264.

Norris, C. (1999). Functional load abdominal training (part 1). Journal of Bodywork and Movement Therapies, 3(3), 150–158. Retrieved from http:// www.physioinfo.co.za/UserFiles/Functional_Load_Abdominal_Training.pdf

O'Sullivan, S., & Siegelman, R. (2010). TherapyEd's national physical therapy examination: Review and study guide. Evanston, IL.

Prentice, W. (1994). Therapeutic modalities in sports medicine (3rd ed.). St. Louis. Mosby.

Rodriguez-Blanco, C. R., Hernandez, J., Algaba, C., Fernandez, M., &De la Quintana, M. (2006). Changes in active mouth opening following a single treatment of latent myofascial trigger points in the masseter muscle involving post-isometric relaxation or strain/counterstrain. Journal of Bodywork and Movement Therapies, 10(3), 197–205. doi:10.1016/j.jbmt.2005.07.002

Schleip, R., Klingler, W., & Lehmann-Horn, F. (2005). Active fascial contractility: Fascia may be able to contract in a smooth muscle-like manner and thereby influence musculoskeletal dynamics. Medical Hypotheses, 65(2), 273–277. doi: 10.1016/j.mehy.2005.03.005

Shah, J., Phillips, T., Danoff, J. V., Gerber, L. H. (2003). A novel microanalytical technique for assaying soft tissue demonstrates significant quantitative biomechanical differences in 3 clinically distinct groups: Normal, latent and active. Archives of Physical Medicine and Research, 84(9), A4.

Simons, D. G., Travell, J. G., & Simons, L. S. (1999). Myofascial pain and dysfunction: The trigger point manual; Upper half of body. (Vol. 1, 2nd ed.). Baltimore: Williams and Wilkins.

Snodgrass, S J. (2002). Thumb pain in physiotherapists: Potential risk factors and proposed prevention strategies. Journal of Manual & Manipulative Therapy, 10(4), 206–217. doi: 10.1179/106698102790819111

Tatom, A. J., & Laman, F. B. (1999). Intertester reliability of identifying strain and counter strain points. Paper presented at the VPTA Annual Conference, Rehabilitation Associates of Central Virginia, Inc. Lynchburg, VA. Retrieved from http://www.jiscs.com/PDFs/AbstractIntertesterReliability.Tatom. Laman.pdf

Travell, J. G., & Simons, D. G. (1983). Myofascial pain and dysfunction: The trigger point manual. Baltimore: Williams and Wilkins.

Upadhyay, S. S., Mullaji, A. B., Luk, K. D. K., & Leong, J. C. Y. (1995). Relation of spinal and thoracic cage deformities and their flexibilities with altered pulmonary functions in adolescent idiopathic scoliosis. Spine, 20(22), 2415–2420.

Voss, D., Ionta, M., & Myers, V. (1985). Proprioceptive neuromuscular facilitation (3rd ed.). Philadelphia: Harper and Row.

Wilson, J. K., Sevier, T. L., Helfst, R. H., Honing, E. W., & Thomann, A. L. (2000). Comparison of rehabilitation methods in the treatment of patellar tendonitis. Journal of Sports Rehabilitation, 9(4), 304-314.

Wu, S.K., Hong, C.Z., You, J.Y, Chen, C.L., Wang, L.H., & Su, F.C.(2009). The kinetic changes of gait across calf myofascial intervention. Paper presented at the ASB 29th Annual Meeting, Cleveland, OH. Retrieved from http://www.asbweb.org/conferences/2005/pdf/0128.pdf

Prime Movers and Range of the Upper Extremity Muscles

Shoulder Flexion
Prime Movers: Anterior deltoid, coracobrachialis
Range: 0 - 180°

Shoulder Extension
Prime Movers: Latissimus dorsi, posterior deltoid
Range: 0 - 45°

Shoulder Adduction
Prime Movers: Pectoralis major, latissimus dorsi
Range: 0 - 40°

Shoulder Abduction
Prime Movers: Middle deltoid, supraspinatus
Range: 0 -180°

Shoulder Internal rotation
Prime Movers: Latissimus dorsi, pectoralis major
Range: 0 - 90°

Shoulder External rotation
Prime Movers: Infraspinatus, teres minor
Range: 0 - 90°

Scapular Elevation
Prime Movers: Trapezius, levator scapulae

Scapular Retraction
Prime Movers: Rhomboid major, rhomboid minor

Scapular Protraction
Prime Movers: Serratus anterior

56

Elbow Flexion
Prime Movers: Brachialis, biceps brachii
Range: 0 - 145°

Elbow Extension
Prime Movers: Triceps brachii
Range: 0 – (-5) °

Forearm Pronation
Prime Movers: Pronator teres, Pronator quadratus
Range: 0 - 90°

Forearm Supination
Prime Movers: Biceps brachii, supinator
Range: 0 - 90°

Wrist Flexion
Prime Movers: Flexor carpi radialis, flexor carpi ulnaris
Range: 0 - 80°

Wrist Extension
Prime Movers: Extensor carpi radialis longus/brevis
Range: 0 -70°

Wrist Abduction
Prime Movers: Extensor carpi radialis longus/brevis
Range: 0 - 20°

Wrist Adduction
Prime Movers: Flexor carpi ulnaris, extensor carpi ulnaris
Range: 0 - 45°[65]

Examination

Upon meeting the Satisfactory Completion Statement, you may receive a certificate of completion at the end of this course.

Contact ceu@rehabsurge.com to find out if this distance learning course is an approved course from your board. Save your course outline and contact your own board or organization for specific filing requirements.

In order to obtain continuing education hours, you must have read the book, have completed the exam and survey. Please include a $10.00 exam fee for your exam. Mail the exam answer sheet and survey sheet to:

Rehabsurge, Inc.

PO Box 287

Baldwin, NY 11510

Allow 2–4 weeks to receive your certificate.

You can also take the exam online at www.rehabsurge.com. Register and pay the exam fee of $10.00. After you passed the exam with a score of 70%, you will be able to print your certificate immediately. See rehabsurge.com for more details.

Exam Questions

1. The first complete publication that talked about the concept of specific trigger points, referred pain and a thorough review of the other published literature was brought out by:

a. Travell and Simons in 1983

b. Hippocrates 400 BC

c. Gorrell in 1983

d. Froriep in the 19th century

2. A condition where pain is caused by a stimulus that does not normally provoke pain is called:

a. Analgesia

b. Allodynia

c. Dysthesia

d. Hyperesthesia

3. A syndrome of sustained burning pain, allodynia and hyperpathia after a traumatic nerve lesion; now classified as complex regional pain syndrome II is:

a. hyperpathia

b. hyperalgesia

c. hypoalgesia

d. causalgia

4. What are mainly composed of certain individual proteins known as myofilaments?

a. fascicles

b. myofibers

c. myofibrils

d. myocytes

5. What is the smallest unit of a muscle or cell? It is the functional unit of length in a muscle.

a. sarcoplasmic retinaculum

b. sarcomere

c. A band

d. I band

6. It is a type of contraction where the practitioner offers a greater counterforce than the patient to lengthen a muscle which is trying to shorten. An example would be controlled micro-trauma.

a. isometric contraction

b. concentric contraction

c. eccentric contraction

d. isokinetic contraction

7. A good example of this law would be the astronauts when they are in space. Because their bones are not subjected to the lines of gravity, they lose bone density.

a. Wolff's law

b. Hooke's law

c. Newton's third law

d. Murphy's law

8. What is the term used to describe pain develops in the joint during myofascial stretching?

a. Referred pain pattern

b. positive stretch sign

c. local twitch reponse

d. limited range of motion

9. This trigger point classification is silent, does not cause spontaneous pain, but is tender upon palpation.

a. active

b. latent

c. satellite

d. central

10. In performing STAR palpation what does "A" stand for?

a. aching

b. active range

c. asymmetry

d. anomaly

11. This palpation technique is when you would grab the affected area with the trigger point in it and hold it. The pinching action is used to apply the pressure. The fibers are pressed between the fingers in a rolling manner while attempting to locate a taut band.

a. flat palpation

b. deep palpation

c. knead palpation

d. pincer palpation

12. Which technique using a solid needle for deactivation and desensitization of a myofascial trigger point which should stimulate a healing response in that tissue and reduce the biomechanical stress of the muscle treated?

a. Local anesthetics

b. Botulinum toxin

c. Dry Needling

d. Transcutaneous Electrical Stimulation

13. All of the following applies to dry needling except:

a. Dry needling assesses and treats myofascial pain due to myofascial trigger points.

b. Dry needling diagnoses and treats several pathological conditions including visceral and systemic dysfunction.

c. Dry needling follows with myofascial stretching exercises.

d.Dry needling use one needle inserted in the myofascial trigger points.

14. This type of stretch requires adopting specific postures based on traditional yoga and maintaining these for some time with deep relaxation breathing. It is a form of self-induced viscoelastic myofascial release.

a. Contract relax antagonist contract

b. hold relax

c. Active isolated stretching

d. Yoga stretching

15. What is stretching by using rapid and bouncing movements? There is a risk of irritation or frank injury.

a. Ballistic stretching

b. Post-isometric relaxation

c. Reciprocal inhibition

d. Proprioceptive neuromuscular facilitation

16. Which type of muscle energy technique is described?

" The shortened muscle is placed midrange position about halfway between a fully stretched and a fully relaxed state. Isometric contraction is performed for 5-10 seconds; while effort is resisted completely. On release, a rapid stretch without bounce is held for 10 seconds. The patient relaxes for 20 seconds. The process is repeated 3-5 times."

a. Postfacilitation stretch method

b. Integrated Neuromuscular Inhibitory Technique

c. Positional Release Technique

d. Active Release Technique

17. Gamma gain appears to represent the amount of muscular activity occurring in the muscular tissue holding the joint in a dysfunctional position. What is the amount of time needed to reset the gamma gain in the muscle?

a. 4 seconds

b. 5 seconds

c. 6 seconds

d. 7 seconds

18. This Ancient East Asian methods make use of any smooth edge, such as buffalo horn or even the metal lid from a jar.

a. Graston

b. Gua Sha

c. ASTYM

d. Accuforce

19. What condition is classified as a patient having at least a 10° lateral curve of the spine for which a recognizable cause is unknown?

a. Spondylosis

b. Idiopathic Scoliosis

c. Ankylosing spondylitis

d. Lumbar Stenosis

20. It is a maneuver that increases the sympathetic outflow to the skeletal muscle when holding one's breath with the glottis closed.

a. induced elevated intrathoracic pressure

b. pressure pain threshold

c. pressure threshold for eliciting referred pain

d. visual analog scale

Answer sheet

Name:_____

Address:_____

Profession:_____

License Number:_____

Date:_____

E-mail Address (optional):_____

Exam:

1.	a	b	c	d
2.	a	b	c	d
3.	a	b	c	d
4.	a	b	c	d
5.	a	b	c	d
6.	a	b	c	d
7.	a	b	c	d
8.	a	b	c	d
9.	a	b	c	d
10.	a	b	c	d
11.	a	b	c	d
12.	a	b	c	d
13.	a	b	c	d
14.	a	b	c	d
15.	a	b	c	d
16.	a	b	c	d
17.	a	b	c	d
18.	a	b	c	d
19.	a	b	c	d
20.	a	b	c	d

Please mail $10.00 and completed form to:

CEU certificate request
Rehabsurge, Inc.
PO Box 287
Baldwin, NY 11510.
Contact Us at:
Phone: +1 (516) 515-1267
Email: ceu@rehabsurge.com

Alternatively, you can take the exam online at **www.rehabsurge.com**
You will receive your certificate instantly.

It is the learner's responsibility to comply with all state and national regulatory board's rules and regulations. This includes but is not limited to:
•verifying and complying with applicable continuing education requirements;
•verifying and complying with all applicable standards of practice;
•verifying and complying with all licensure requirements;
•any other rules or laws identified in the learners state or regulatory board that is not mentioned here.
It is the learner's responsibility to complete ALL coursework in order to receive credit. This includes but is not limited to:
•Reading all course materials fully;
•Completing all course activities to meet the criteria set forth by the instructor;
•Completing and passing all applicable tests and quizzes. All learner's MUST take a comprehensive online exam where they MUST get at least 70%. Getting 70% is a requirement to pass.

IMPORTANT: Rehabsurge reserves the right to deny continuing education credits or withdraw credits issued at any time if: Coursework is found to be incomplete; It is determined that a user falsified, copied, and/or engaged in any flagrant attempt to manipulate, modify, or alter the coursework just to receive credit; and/or It is determined that the coursework was not completed by the user.

If any of the conditions above are determined, Rehabsurge reserves the right to notify any applicable state and national boards along with supporting documentation.

Program Evaluation Form

Rehabsurge, Inc. works to develop new programs based on your comments and suggestions, making your feedback on the program very important to us. We would appreciate you taking a few moments to evaluate this program.

Course Start Date:_____   Course End Date: _____

Course Start Time:_____   Course End Time:_____

Identity Verification: Name:_____

Profession:_____ License Number:_____State: _____

Please initial to indicate that you are the individual who read the book and completed the test.

Initial here:_____

May we use your comments and suggestions in upcoming marketing materials.   Yes   No

Would you take another seminar from Rehabsurge, Inc.?   Yes   No

The educational level required to read the book is: Beginner   Intermediate   Advanced

The course is:	(5-Yes/Excellent)			(1- No/Poor)	
Relevant to my profession	5	4	3	2	1
Valuable to my profession	5	4	3	2	1
Content matched stated objectives	5	4	3	2	1
Complete coverage of materials	5	4	3	2	1
Teaching ability	5	4	3	2	1
Organization of material	5	4	3	2	1
Effective	5	4	3	2	1

Please rate the objectives. After reading the material, how well do you feel you are able to meet:

Objective 1	5	4	3	2	1
Objective 2	5	4	3	2	1
Objective 3	5	4	3	2	1
Objective 4	5	4	3	2	1
Objective 5	5	4	3	2	1

What was the most beneficial part of the program? What was the least beneficial part of the program? _____
_____

What would you like to see added to the program? In what ways might we make this program experience better for you?_____
_____

If you have any general comments on this topic or program please explain.

_____
_____

Please tell us what other programs or topics might interest you?

_____
_____

Thank you for participating and taking the time to join us today!

9805545R00043

Printed in Great Britain
by Amazon.co.uk, Ltd.,
Marston Gate.